PRAISE FOR

Pearls of Wisdom, Pure & Powerful

"You rarely find words like *love, prayer, tears, heart, spirit* and *intuition* in success literature these days. But you'll find them in here! Along with *empowered, passion, balance* and *certainty.* Discover that real success lies within." ~ William D. Esteb – Chiropractic patient and advocate since 1981, www.patientmedia.com.

"Knowing Dr. Liz and many of the contributing authors of this book, I knew this book would be filled with the wisdom of those who have reached within themselves and touched the source of infinite possibilities – which is indeed the source of all. As I started reviewing the various contributions, I was inspired by the clarity and certainty each of these pure and powerful woman expresses in describing their journey towards living an innately guided life. The wisdom within these pages, when applied, will transform lives. Those who read this book and apply its wisdom will touch and release the innate giant within and discover the life of their dreams that has been within them since they were loved into existence. This book offers to all who integrate its wisdom into their being, the pure and powerful life that living innately provides." ~ Dr. Peter Amlinger – International Speaker, coach and 2007 Canadian Chiropractor of the Year.

"Simply inspiring – a magnificent chiropractic gem!" ~ Dr. John Demartini – Founder of the Demartini Institute™, Best-selling author of *Count Your Blessings – The Healing Power of Gratitude and Love,* Featured in "The Secret".

"The Innate wisdom of this book propels people into action and is a timeless gift for all chiropractors!" ~ International Health Publishing.

"Relevant and reflective, refreshing and purposeful, encouraging and uplifting for all our souls!" ~ Becky Halstead – Retired US Army Brigadier General, fibromyalgia chiropractic patient, Spokesperson for the Foundation for Chiropractic Progress.

"An enlightening work of experiences for new and existing Chiropractors and new business owners in the health professions, reminding us to think and feel with our internal wisdom." ~ Karen Furneaux MSc. – Kinesiology & Sport Psychology, President & CEO Promise Performance, Inc., 3-time Olympian, 2-time World Champion, 17-year member Canadian Sprint Kayak Team.

"Wow! It turns out that *Pearls of Wisdom, Pure and Powerful* is not just another sound-good title for a book. It is an accurate compendium of the shared warm, personal stories, incredible understanding, knowledge and insights of 19 of our profession's most successful and enlightened female Chiropractors. Together, they say it all - vividly displaying their individual journeys on the way to establishing the incredible belief systems and love that have turned them into true healers and advocates of our precious Chiropractic Principles. This is a MUST read for every female chiropractor in the world and their male counterparts, as well." ~ Larry Markson DC – *The Markson Connection / The Cabin Experience.*

"A brilliant compilation of the female leaders in chiropractic, so much to be said, so little time to say it." ~ Dr. Jim Sigafoose – recognized worldwide for his inspirational messages, Chiropractic Philosophy and legendary teachings.

"This is a book of rare grace. The authors reveal in their stories the most profound depths of the feminine qualities that are so necessary, at least in part, in the health practitioner-empathy, compassion, sensitivity, intuition, and yes, humour and intelligence. These women live in authentic harmony with the life force, flowing freely, and they guide us to practice in this rewarding way." ~ Dr. Judy Hinwood – Mentor Emeritus, *The Centre for Powerful Practices*, Casuarina Beach, Australia.

"Amazing things happen in chiropractic when you are in tune with innate, on focus, and accept cases where you know that the removal of nerve pressure can enable all types of healing miracles to take place in the human body. This is a book of inspiration." ~ Dr John Hinwood – "The Miracle Man", Casuarina Beach, Australia, author of international best seller *You Can Expect a Miracle.*

"The idea of women sharing with individuals of like-mind and talent was BRILLIANT. Some stories made me smile while others made me (temporarily) sad; but they all made me proud to be associated with so many fine women in such an amazing profession. Common threads were noted running through every story regardless of the choice of college, technique and any presenting circumstance. Bottom line - we must not only live consciously but also with Passion and Purpose." ~ Dr. Maxine McMullen – Internationally known educator and professor in pediatrics, Founder of the ICA's Pediatric Diplomate program.

"The women leaders of Chiropratic stepped to the plate and hit a home run with *Pearls of Wisdom, Pure & Powerful* – their message is a must read by not only Chiropractors, but anyone seeking wisdom about the game of life." ~ Kenneth C. Thomas BS, MS, DC, CCSP – International Speaker, Vice President of Academics Parker College of Chiropractic.

"These inspirational stories are brilliant, like diamonds! What an honour to read the words of these astounding Chiropractors." ~ Dr. Tracy Kennedy-Shanks – 4th Generation chiropractor with first family visit to a chiropractor in 1906; Toowoomba, Australia.

"With pride and confidence I can say, that if the women who authored this book ruled our world, there would be global peace, health and harmony. Their stories deeply moved me. Thank you. Thank you for gracefully and with conviction putting into words what I do, what I say, and what I feel every day in my Practice. I am absolutely honoured to be one of you!" ~ Dr. Rosemary Emily Oman – Switzerland.

"Compelling reading from a great wellspring of untapped potential – the women of chiropractic have something significant to say, and they say it in *Pearls of Wisdom*!"
~ Dennis Perman DC – co-founder of The Masters Circle.

"*Pearls of Wisdom* is filled with incredible gifts of insight from many talented and wise people. No matter what type of wisdom you are seeking - health, life or other, you will find many inspiring pearls in this book and you will refer to it throughout your lifetime." ~ Dr. Eric Plasker – CEO The Family Practice, Inc., Best Selling Author, *The 100 Year Lifestyle™*.

"This book will inspire you. It is packed with timeless lessons and Principles and is a must read for every woman in the profession. Dr. Liz has put together a wonderful collection of experiences and pearls of wisdom from some of the most exceptional women in chiropractic. I am fortunate to know, and have grown to love Dr. Liz and many of the contributing authors. Well done Dr. Liz and friends, this work is a great example of your continuing contribution to humanity."
~ Dr. James Carter, DC – Personal Development Specialist, Australia.

"I have known Dr. Liz Anderson-Peacock as a colleague and friend for many years, and the quality of my life has been greatly enhanced through her work and her wisdom. *Pearls of Wisdom* is brilliant, because she is. She shares her love of life and Universal Principles like no other. Read this book and be inspired to discover true health. By knowing, you will receive the gift of free will and personal choice." ~ Dr. Gilles LaMarche – author, speaker and Vice President Parker College of Chiropractic.

"If I was not already a Chiropractor I would go back to school to become one! The strength and dedication of these amazing women is inspiring beyond words — I have never been so proud to be a chiropractor. I can only hope that their extraordinary stories will empower others to have such purpose and passion for chiropractic in order for us to leave a great legacy to humanity." ~ Nathalie Beauchamp B.Sc., DC – Co-Author of the book *Wellness On The Go.*

Pearls of Wisdom, Pure & Powerful

Dr. Liz Anderson-Peacock

INTERNATIONAL HEALTH PUBLISHING

www.InternationalHealthPublishing.com

www.pearlsofwisdompandp.com

INTERNATIONAL HEALTH PUBLISHING
February 22, 2008
Publishing Group Affirming Truth & Innate Wisdom

First International Health Publishing trade paperback edition August 2010

For information about special discounts for bulk purchase, please contact International Health Publishing at writer@InternationalHealthPublishing.com.

International Health Publishing can bring authors to your live events. For more information or to book an event, contact writer@InternationalHealthPublishing.com or for more information visit our website: www.InternationalHealthPublishing.com.

Pearls Of Wisdom, Pure & Powerful
Dr. Liz Anderson-Peacock
www.pearlsofwisdompandp.com

ISBN-13 978-0-9818353-5-8
ISBN-10 0-9818353-5-X

Library of Congress Control Number: 2010930749

SAN 856-6925

Manufactured in the United States of America, and printed on the finest 100% postconsumer-waste recycled paper

10 9 8 7 6 5 4 3 2 1

Dedication

This book is foremost dedicated to prospective students, females, and future Chiropractors.

This book is dedicated to our Vitalistic brothers and sisters, our colleagues preceding us, who provided an opportunity and a 'place' for us. With a *will* based upon solid Principles and Universal Laws, they paved the way for our profession beginning at odds to the prevailing thoughts of the time.

This book is dedicated to those who continue in the trenches today making a difference one life at a time, colleagues in and out of practice, women creating innovative practices, chiropractors reaching out to the masses to teach and adjust.

This book is dedicated to the indelible impressions made upon us by the men in our lives: fathers, mentors, colleagues, friends, brothers and sons. We learn from you every day. When we meet you on a soul level, the soul knows no gender.

Acknowledgements

We are eternally grateful to the many Chiropractors preceding us, who in the earlier times often faced very difficult circumstances. Thankfully they did not give up. Some were jailed to defend a different way of thinking. Some women became doctors before women were even emancipated and allowed to vote.

Behind any success is a team of dedicated individuals. All of the contributing writers to this book are successful colleagues, and I thank them for their time and energy. More importantly, they are friends who I could call-on at any time for help. If they could not be there personally, they would find an alternate, a resource or even the words or phrase to move me along.

At heart, these colleagues have a passion to give, to serve and to heal. They are remarkable women who truly did not have the time to add "yet one more thing" in their busy schedules. As one said, *"If what I write makes a difference to even just one woman, then it is worth it."* At their core, these Doctors hold a value of loving service and practice the service of loving. They are dedicated to making a difference in the world and share with you their combined experience of *over 400 years of clinical life*!

I thank each author for diligently writing and sharing their story. I am truly blessed to have you as friends.

I also thank our very helpful publisher, Dr. Lizie Pilicy and *International Health Publishing*. She is also a Doctor of Chiropractic, as well as an elite soccer player. I do not know how she finds the time to juggle her publishing company with her practice; she too has a remarkable story.

I wish to thank my husband, Barry, who constantly reminds me of what is important. I also thank my family for providing a base of never-ending support during some very challenging times. Thank you Dr. Tom, Dr. Andrea, Chris, Dee Dee and Carrie. I also thank many dear friends and colleagues, and you know who you are; and for fear of missing one, I provide a general thank you.

We all have mentors and people who have profoundly influenced us, and are eternally grateful for their caring and guidance.

Contents

Pearls of Wisdom, Pure & Powerful

Foreword

Innate intelligence knows more in one second than you can
ever know.
~ B.J. Palmer

Why an Oyster and Pearl on the cover? The formation of a
natural pearl begins when a foreign substance slips into an
oyster between the mantle and the shell, irritating the
mantle. It is somewhat like the oyster getting a splinter. The
oyster's innate response is to protect itself by walling-off the
irritant. It adapts by enveloping the irritant with layers of
the same substance used to create the shell. This process
eventually forms a pearl. So, a priceless gem, a pearl arises
as a result of an uncomfortable stress an oyster overcomes.

This process is analogous to our lives, since life presents
invariable irritations as we experience, adapt, change and
integrate our world. From this we grow as human beings.
We learn more from mistakes than from what we know. We
implement what we think we know, and observe the
resulting effect. Through living we gain wisdom. We are each
unique and need to express and celebrate our uniqueness. No
one else walks this earth as you. Just as pearls, people posses
a variety of characteristics. Crises create opportunity for us
to stretch and create something new – just as an oyster
creates a pearl.

Pearls of Wisdom, Pure & Powerful was conceived at the end of March 2010. I sent a thought into the Universe on how phenomenal workingwomen could feel more connected to others and to themselves. Our technology is connecting us more than ever; however, there is less emotional connection and support. We speak less often, we share less than we used to, and only in sound bites. We read headlines and summaries. Technology makes us run at full-speed at all times. We feel obligated to always be on the go, and have no excuses for less than full throttle. We may communicate more often, but about less and less important things – reality television shows, fashion trends, latest fads, negative news; but what about *real* connection?

What is important to you? Why did you enter into your profession? What do you love about it? What do you value? When was the last time you wrote yourself a "thank you" letter? When was the last time you reassessed your vocation and how your practice reflects your values? Or does it?

When I ask my clients to define the difference between what they *do* and who they *are*, they are perplexed by the question. We seem to define ourselves more and more by what we do and what we have accomplished. If what you *do* was eliminated, how would your definition of *self* be impacted? Would you characterize yourself differently?

I have recently had the experience of change within my own life, and one of the gifts has been for me to become reacquainted with the essence of who I am.

Are we limiting ourselves to what we think we "ought to" act or look like? Or rather, are we expressing our inborn potential through our art and styles of practice, through our communication in how we listen, teach and mentor? Are we following the guidance of our intuition?

The collaborating writers within *Pearls of Wisdom, Pure & Powerful* have had very different experiences within our profession, each finding a uniquely fitting path to follow.

Everyone has a story to tell, and the significance of sharing the tales of our experience comes with the lessons learned. Stories connect people, provide insight; they make us smile, laugh and cry. Through telling stories of our experience, we share our journey in life together, allowing us to come to know one another just a little more intimately.

The Birth Of A Book

At the end of March 2010, an email invitation to be a part of the creation of this book was forwarded to twenty-five women Chiropractors possessing a great deal of practice experience. They were allotted thirty-days to write approximately ten pages on one or a combination of three story topics: a poignant patient story; why they entered into a Vitalistic Profession; and/or to share a valuable piece of knowledge they learned through practicing – knowledge potentially helpful for other women and Chiropractors.

With the time and topic parameters required for involvement, six women responded by saying they would like to participate, but given their present situation could not meet the time-lines. For those that did not participate, I appreciated the boundaries they set for themselves; as for many females, we have challenges in saying "No."

This book does not purport to represent all of the exceptional women in our field, although, there were a few qualifying characteristics considered for participation. Chief distinctions included experience in practice, with representation of a Vitalistic practice-style – meaning those that teach and live the Principles as taught by our founders. The truth in why we deliver a Chiropractic adjustment is extremely significant to us. We teach the basics, the supremacy and integrative qualities of the nervous system as the master controlling system of the body. Interference within the nervous system, direct or indirect, changes the potential for natural communication within the body.

The doctors contributing to this manuscript have oodles of life experience. No doubt we all have faced the challenges that come with running and managing a practice: fear, doubt, rejection, hurt, embarrassment and humility. On the flip side, we also have experienced the fulfillment our vocation offers: joy, opportunity, reward, connection, nurturing, and miracles. Not to say these are lessons learned from reading about them in a book or hearing about them in a lecture, but instead through first-hand life experience.

These women talk and live congruent Principles, and are consistent on and off the stage. Our contributions are the essence of who we are, and putting our best efforts forward, how we try to live. Just as any human, we have our own flaws, moments of struggle, and are presented with new lessons in life. Not everything is easy. During the times when we may not have been living in harmony, we express the feelings associated with friction, and how we eventually returned onto a path of purpose.

We made mistakes, stood-up to unanticipated adversity, and at times, steered through 180° turns. We learned and grew. We became stronger. Our conquests contribute to a collective wisdom. Our hope is to assist you in growth. It matters not if you are a prospective student, a graduate, a veteran, a Chiropractor, or even an electrician. Upon reading this book, one could literally replace and re-insert the title of any profession. The lessons are not limited to one profession or one group of women, but universal to all.

Continually, the contributing writers donate countless hours of time on behalf of our Chiropractic profession: conference calls, in-person meetings, association meetings discussing directions of regulations, associations, educational requirements, seminar preparations, mentoring... the list goes on. They are involved and speaking their voices, displaying attributes for making a difference. When not directly involved, then supporting someone with similar values is an equally valuable contribution. Support comes in many forms and women are masters at collaborative efforts.

Giving It Up To The Universe

This book is a reflection of what I ultimately envisioned and sent into the Universe. When the original idea came to me, I inherently knew the contributors would triumph with their stories illustrating commonalities logically strung together as one. I trusted the loose style of my email request to be enough to arouse a naturally-right flow.

As women, we speak through our emotional experience. Even with all we may *cognitively* know, we do not change until we *feel* it. Knowledge is valuable, but until we are moved or touched by something or someone, we usually do not change. When we *feel* it, it becomes us.

As doctors, we are only too often in our heads; yet as facilitators of healing, are more dynamic when in our hearts. We share our practices and real life moments with you. We know you have similar experiences. Data and information without experience is merely philosophy; but when we have a personal experience it becomes real and part of our life. We are changed, we learn, we integrate, and we become wiser.

Others Want To Hear Your Voice

While speaking at the Canadian Association of Family Enterprises (CAFE) meeting about family business hosted at our office, I realized our job is not to make the next generation's life easier *per se*, but perhaps to provide a future with greater opportunity to excel in ways we can only dream of now. As we have benefitted from those before us, we are planting seeds for those that follow. As a result, many are flying further, faster and earlier then us. I cannot imagine a better profession to enter into as a woman, and we hope this book will help you along your journey.

Many of the contributing authors mentor, some additionally coach, so please know we hear and truly understand the challenges expressed by our "sisters." We invite you into our world and appreciate you, as we are a reflection of you and you of us.

At the end of the book, there are several engaging assignments. Specifically, the assignment called *"Applying the Bullets to Your Life"* to use for your own self-study by correlating the bullet points highlighted at the end of each chapter. We hope this book creates a connection from one to another, and look forward to *Volume II*.

Welcome & Enjoy,

Dr. Liz

Once you get the big idea, all else follows.
~ *B.J. Palmer*

1

Response Ability
Dr. Liz Anderson-Peacock

I remember the day I "discovered" Chiropractic. It was life changing. During my years in university, I watched many friends go into their respective fields after two years of "pre-whatever." Dentistry, medicine, and law were the common ones. I was unsure what I would do after earning my Bachelor of Science, but decided I would finish the program to buy time for choosing my career.

At that time, I knew three people who entered a profession called *Chiropractic.* I had never heard of a Chiropractor. I had no idea what they did, but was curious. When my friends and I reunited after their first year in their programs, the medical students looked *spent,* complained of exhaustion, hair loss, ulcers and many were taking multiple meds. In contrast, the Chiropractic students, though tired from the rigorous hours of academics, were generally more excited about life, could hardly wait to explain how the body functions and to apply their newly learned knowledge. They wanted to palpate landmarks on people. They wanted to see and experience people. It struck me as peculiar, since both of the professions had similar academic studies in the first year. I assumed it was due to the culture of how things were taught through the institutions. Their personas' made an indelible impression on me.

As I continued through university, I was drawn to study anatomy. In my fourth year, I enrolled in a comparative anatomy course and an anatomy of mammals course. Both involving anatomical drawings of my dissections, along with the interplay of comparing structure and function. In my fourth year working a summer job with parks and recreation in Alberta, I hurt my low back and went to my first Chiropractic appointment.

So I went to a Chiropractor: Dr. Judy Forrester in Calgary. She asked me about my history, and while performing an examination, checked my full spine. While palpating my neck, she inquired about sinus problems, allergies, stuffy nose, watery eyes and asked if I experienced any symptoms.

To make a long story short, I experienced severe environmental allergies as a child, endured ten years of allergy shots and multiple medications. I remember back to the age of five chewing *Allerest, Dimetapp* or *Pyribenzamine* before swallowing with a glass of water. I had an air purifier in my bedroom. My family resided on a beautiful fresh water lake in Barrie, Ontario. I was a very enthusiastic and active *tomboy*, and loved to swim and play outdoors. Suffering from allergies began every year in June and continued through the first frost.

So Dr. Judy's question struck me as interesting. Since I had been taking the medications, I assumed all was well within. I appreciated the break from symptoms the meds provided so I could continue on with life. When she asked, I remember thinking, "What does my neck have to do with allergies?"

The Chiropractor asked me the cause of my allergies, and I made the standard reply, "Primarily dust, molds, dander and pollens."

She asked, "Why?"

I replied, "Because my body is releasing too much histamine when exposed to allergens."

She asked, "Why is your body making too much histamine?"

I gave a circular reply, "Because it is reacting to the pollens, dust, dander and mold."

Realizing I was not understanding her point, she changed her line of questioning and asked, "If you and I are breathing the same air, wouldn't we both be breathing air with the same pollens?"

I nodded a yes.

"If you and I are breathing the same pollens in the air, then shouldn't we both be having the same response *if* the allergens were the *true* cause of allergies?"

I had no answer. I thought my symptoms were due to allergens and by taking drugs and allergy shots the problem would resolve. I never thought to ask why my body was doing something different than other people. I had never considered asking or looking at how other people may have been living their lives differently from me.

She then explained the modulating effect of the nervous system on the immune system, and how they communicate with one other. She said I likely had an *insult* in my neck at some point in my past, impacting my body's ability to adapt to the environment. My body was responding, but not appropriately for the situation.

I went home and asked my mother about the possibility of a childhood trauma, and she noted that I experienced two black eyes during a car accident at around age two. No seatbelt laws in those days, and I was in the front seat. The collision caused me to fly out of the seat and hit the dashboard headfirst. I was checked-out by doctors and told I was fine, although my mother does not remember my neck being checked.

In consideration of Dr. Judy's proposition of a childhood trauma causing insult to my neck, I thought back to my younger years. I used to see how many steps I could jump inflight down the stairs in my house. Most of the time I landed on the pillows – the operative word being 'most.' Also, there were the bicycle wrecks: riding into the side of the house multiple times because I did not know how to use the brakes, or the time a stick was caught in the spokes of my front wheel and I fell on my face chipping a tooth. I played sports, fell out of trees, and so on; pick one incident, they were all physically traumatic.

To Change Others Worlds, First Change Yourself

I retuned to Dr. Judy's office and had my first adjustment and my world changed. My low back was not nearly as important to me as resolving my allergies. Of course, at first I did not fully grasp the importance of rest and diet. I did not yet understand how they affected the chemistry within my body, particularly the excitability of my neuro-immune system. But, upon my first adjustment, my allergies improved immediately by about 75-80 percent. I stopped the drugs; I stopped the allergy shots, and felt like I had a new found life. As if someone removed earmuffs from my ears and the fog clouding my brain, I felt able to process information faster, and with greater clarity and integration.

The following fall semester I entered Chiropractic as a career.

Without A Plan

Upon graduating from Chiropractic school, I was without a plan. I fell back on some opportunities, but in retrospect I had not fully prepared myself for the work required to begin a practice. I thought, like many, I would graduate and people would just start pouring into my office for care. I thought the *hard part* (school) was over. What a wake up call.

I began what I referred to as my 'default practice' in a location and a city I was not fond of. A smarter person would have asked "Why?" Sometimes the things we need to learn are so apparent to others, but in the moment not to ourselves. Practice was slow, arduous and I was depressed. I had done well in school, yet in my first practice felt like an utter failure. I had never envisioned I would experience complications starting out. Everything seemed so difficult. I worked long hours and commuted a great distance for a number of months. I woke up at 4:30 AM and returned home by 9:30 PM. In retrospect, if I had a patient working those hours five and a half days a week including Saturday mornings, I would have said it was unsustainable over time.

When the winter came, I moved closer to the office. But still, I muscled through every moment. I was not congruent with what I advised to patients, not eating well nor living well. In the morning, I grabbed coffee and something with high sugar content to stimulate my energy. By the time I returned home in the evening, I was no longer hungry; if I ate it kept me awake later. I was in the vicious cycle of being too tired for physical activity, and made the clichéd excuse of 'not having enough time' to exercise. I was so unhappy and heading in a downward spiral.

At the end of one day, I remember sitting by my bookshelf seeing a piece of paper between two books. I pulled it out, an essay I wrote prior to school on why I wanted to become a Chiropractor. "To change lives, to make a difference, to be of service, to use my brain and physical skills." My eyes welled-up in disappointed with myself. I felt deep sadness and embarrassment. I sat blaming everyone else, shifting the responsibility elsewhere, not yet accepting it as my own. I remember thinking I would just leave the profession and do something else; that it was not for me. I almost did. I knew something needed to change. Not long after that evening, I began to realize it was *me.*

There Are No Failures, Only Lessons

About the same time as my practice seemed to be failing, my intimate relationship with a colleague was failing. Neither of us was happy. I am sure I contributed mostly to our dismay, as I was so miserable I didn't even want to be around myself. So I relished in my 'pauvre moi' attitude, repelling most everyone around me.

The pivotal decision to leave that practice, the relationship, my house, and to move was instrumental for my future growth. By no means was it easy, though. I remember packing and traveling 'home' to the town where I grew up, the same town my parents retired back to. My move back home was the sort of retreat with one's tail between their legs, very humbling and with feelings of inadequacy. My parents showed nothing less than loving support, and had more confidence in me than I did in myself. All I knew, I was starting over. Moving forward on my own, I created a sink or swim situation: no one to rescue me, my outcome fully dependent upon me. Unknowingly at that time, I was creating a springboard for my future.

After my move, I reconnected with former Chiropractic classmates, who loved what they were doing in their practices. I asked them what they had done to help themselves in practice. They noted, "The Carter Program." I asked what it entailed, and they said I just had to experience it.

I remember receiving the registration material and thinking I could not afford the fees. In deep thought, I recognized that what I was enduring *had* to be more painful than change. Knowing I did not want to repeat what I had preciously created, I needed to do something drastically different. Sometimes we change when the pain of the same becomes greater than the pain of change, and that was my primary motivator to join the program.

Unaware of the synchronicity, I listened to a cassette tape series: "You See It When You Believe It," by Dr. Wayne Dyer. Parts of the series hit me like a ton of bricks. My paraphrased memory of his words resonate, "Why worry about things you can change, because if you *can* change them then just change them." Furthermore, "Why worry about things you cannot change, because if you cannot control them in any way, let them go." Simple to say, difficult to do, yet the concept encouraged me then, and carries with me still.

Anew in my hometown, I began reorganizing my life. I introduced myself to local colleagues. Two said, "Don't come here, it is pretty full," implying the city reached a saturation of Chiropractors. There were about eight or nine at the time. The others embraced me with open arms. I thought, "Humm, interesting," making a mental note of the two with a *scarcity* complex.

I was granted a bank loan – but only with the co-signing of a *male.* Although very thankful to my father for co-signing, I wondered if the same would have been required if I was male. It only fed my determination. I made my own bench tables and upholstered them myself, acquired used office furniture, then hired an assistant – the small business grant affording the initial months of her employment.

I opened my small practice and attended my first Carter Program. Formidable, it addressed full-on responsibility, commitment and accountability in everything we think, say and do. The top three 'take home lessons' from the program included:

1. Practice reflects me, and professional growth is in accordance to personal growth.

2. If I do not like an outcome, I change something; only I can foster change, no one else.

3. Practice is about being of service to patients first. Meet them where *they are*; listen, educate, provide choices and guidance. Service to others always comes first. Everything you think, say and do is intended as benefit.

At times, we have all been in circumstances of absolute frustration, fear and despair. I testify I would not change one part of this process, for the lessons promoted my growth.

Responsibility On A New Level

I learned responsibility is a duty first to oneself to commit fully to what one says one will do, and having the discipline to live by one's word. Responsibility makes us trustworthy, reliable and solid. Responsibility means when one commits to something or someone, it is seen through. If things should drastically change and a commitment is broken, then one is upfront and honest to modify the agreement.

The change I yearned for presented within each part of my day. Implementing organizational procedures, I reduced my hours, served more people, attended seminars and still had time to read and exercise. Within six months, I developed my practice to its full capacity, which has been maintained throughout my career. I met wonderful like-minded colleagues and we gathered for philosophical discussions. To gain clarity, we asked why we do what we do? We had regular mastermind meetings, challenging each other to be better, to serve in more ways. As I grew, so did my practice. I am grateful to Jim Carter and remember fondly and cherish the colleagues I met during the 'Carter Days.'

Ask For Help And It Will Appear

I was delivered into a higher sphere of influence. My study of the works by Dr. John Demartini in the latter part of the Eighties continued to expand my mind: Breakthrough, quantum healing, spiritual healing, speed-reading. I attended DE's in Atlanta, Sigafoose's Gathering, "Little Crow," also known as Ron Gentry. Gentry was an apprentice to an elder in the Choctaw tribe, and lead me through arrowhead and Native American teachings.

Each of my breakthroughs connected me more intimately with my heart and intuition, guiding me towards yet more lessons for growth. Over this time, I met my current husband Barry, who continues to offer great influence in my life.

When I was the ready student, the teachers appeared. In the early Nineties, I started attending Seminars, such as Total Solutions, Pure and Powerful, and have continued regular attendance at Parker Seminars since 1990. The seminars I attended early on in my career were most impressionable. Without question, I admit any seminar could have inspired the creative change needed within me. I eagerly ran after my dreams and the vision of my practice.

Passion For People, Profession And Principle

The combination of the colleagues I spent time with and the seminars I attended filled my heart and stirred a serious passion to serve my community, as well as the profession. While also being very serious, I certainly have fun while serving both.

My vocation exists due to my community – specifically, the patients I serve daily. I offer gratitude to patients and the community at large for their support and for providing a wonderful lifestyle and surrounding environment for living. With thanks I give back, maintaining the flow and balance of what comes in with what goes out. If I covet what comes in, the Universal Principle of motion is broken. As B.J. Palmer said, "Motion is Life and Life is Motion." His thought applies on both a macroscopic and quantum level. Involvement with supporting groups and charities is one way to complete the cycle of giving and receiving.

The ability to practice relies heavily upon governing bodies and associations. In support of the growth of my profession, I am compelled to serve on a variety of committees as opportunity arises. I feel strongly about stepping forward to serve on behalf of a cause greater than myself.

A profession is a reflection of those within it, every voice and opinion matters. Each quantifiably adds up to determine the *tone* and direction of a profession. We are carrying a torch from forefathers before us, persecuted and jailed merely because they were Chiropractors. What if *they* gave up on their ideals, or allowed their Principles to be over ruled by the masses? Where would we be today?

Sitting on numerous boards and committees in many ways has been an eye opener, providing visibility of the various schools of thought. I have gained appreciation of others' perspectives, even if I may not fully agree with them.

Within our profession exists a remarkable breadth and depth to naturally attract different populations of people. The organizing Principles of D.D. Palmer, B.J. Palmer, and Stephenson lay our ground. Fundamentally, we are based on a Vitalistic model. The daily practice and application of the Laws of Life and Vitalistic Universal Principles distinguish Chiropractic within the field of health care. Our celebration comes with being able to maintain our uniqueness to manifest a divine shift in flow of current health systems.

To understand how we have been delivered to where we are today, and to connect with our pioneers, I joined groups with a long list of our professions' historical figures. I met some really old, old-timers and felt blessed to break bread with them, hearing their stories before they passed.

Now, I realize sitting on committees or serving in elected offices is not for everyone. There are many ways to serve and make an impact. Being supportive of like-minded individuals, attending meetings, asking questions, donating to schools, research groups, and other similarly resonating organizations are all models of service. When financially supporting a group, you have the right to ask questions, as you are a co-partner, on some level. Invariably, when one asks a question, others are wondering the same thing. Posing and answering questions creates clarity.

> Whatever you can do or dream you can, begin it. Boldness
> has genius, power and magic in it!
> ~ *John Anster*, in a 'very free' translation of Faust from
> 1835

In practice, when I kept rooted in our philosophy and talked the 'TIC,' I saw miracles; if I strayed or began to coast, I did not. In accordance with the founding Principles, I asked patients why they lived the way they lived, and what they thought about how they lived their lives. I asked them to consider if there might be better ways. I asked them to connect with their feelings and become aware of their body through the course of their day. I invited them to be accountable for their life, how they were living, and to spend time in it. If they did not like their results, I asked them to use themselves as their own experiment to monitor change.

I asked patients where they would rank themselves on a sliding scale ranging from death to super-ideal health. I asked them what they needed to do to move in the direction they wanted. We created baby steps for their success, and of course revisited and adjusted accordingly. This created freedom for me in practice, and placed the responsibility of health squarely on patients. In addition to locating and correcting areas of interference with their bodies, my job was to teach patients about the Principles and the supremacy of the nervous system, and support them in making changes.

Some were ready and some were not. Those that were, prepared and took action; those not ready were pretty much upfront about it. Some had no idea change was needed; but when presented, they became curious and asked questions.

In Life, To Each Their Own Path – Celebrate It

Every one of us is on a path. The illuminated path reveals itself in different ways. When an opportunity presents itself, we may or may not feel prepared. We may be focused on evolving in one area of our life and not in others. Transformation is not a linear process. There is a common tendency to revert back to old habits, falling into the comfortable and familiar. Neither good nor bad, it just is. I see my job as creating opportunity and providing inspiration for people to evoke positive change along their path.

Continue Being A Student In Life

For me, I know when I am not adapting; I feel restless and stagnant. In stagnation, I become complacent, a bit bored and dull. My inner light does not shine as brightly. I like to continually be learning and I love a challenge. I have encountered this restlessness a few times in my career, and it has one way or another caused upheavals as well as pleasant alterations.

When I developed a very successful practice in serving patients and enjoying them, I wondered if there was more 'out there' for me. I had some remarkable experiences with children teaching me yet another dimension of Chiropractic and healing. I considered entering (at that time) the only available Pediatric Diplomat program available, offered through the cooperation of Palmer and the ICA. Since its inception, Chiropractic has always served children and pregnant moms-to-be, though before the early Nineties not many formal diplomats or academic programs focused on mothers and children. Palmer and the ICA began their Pediatric Diplomat in 1994.

I flew from Toronto to Chicago thirty times over three years, and eventually earned the Diplomat in Chiropractic Pediatrics. With application of my newly learned knowledge to practical experiences with patients, I was intellectually stimulated. Although I had not planned it, my interest in pediatrics eventually opened doors to opportunities with numerous groups. Expanding my practice into the areas of prenatal and pediatric care shifted my practice into what I call a 'generations practice.' Multiple generations of families saw us as their primary healthcare provider.

I remember my eyes flooding with tears when a mother with a wonderful family reminisced on how their oldest daughter had poor confidence in school. The daughter's teacher predicted she might not make it through high school, advising the family not to expect much from her. I wondered, what kind of person does that – thinking they can determine a child or any other human being's potential from their limited point of view? From a Chiropractic perspective, her daughter's upper cervical spine was very subluxated. The mother remembered my encouraging words for her daughter. I said, although I did not know her abilities, I *did* know she was put on this earth for a reason and she needed to find out what it was, then go for it. Further, I explained the interference in her upper neck could be choking her potential or clouding her from her purpose, confusing her. If the interference is removed, the ability of her body to function would improve. With the first adjustments, she remembers her life changing. Her academic marks improved, as did her self-esteem. She is a remarkable lady.

The same mother also had two other children, the youngest borne while she was under Chiropractic care throughout the pregnancy. One day in passing, the mother mentioned that her youngest said, "I know if anything ever happens and I can not get home, I can go to Dr. Liz for help." I was deeply touched by a child's trust in me.

In practice, there have been many days of eyes welling up with the stories people share. As Chiropractors, we care for the *person* with the *body*, rather than the other way around. Providing a safe environment within a community is large part of practice, and is reflected by patients' trust in us.

Unconditionally Loving Our Patients

Sometimes we need to unconditionally love our patients when they do not love themselves. We need to give them hope and see their potential. This begins with unconditionally loving our self, and attending to our own needs outside the office in order to be able to serve within it. We need to appreciate all sides of ourselves – all shades, positives and negatives, and respect both. How could we help others and be fully present if they push our buttons for our own needs? People come to us and our responsibility is to be fully present for them. To be fully present we need to train ourselves to focus on being in the present-time whenever we are with another. This is central to what we do, as a moment feels like an eternity when someone is truly *with* us. In that moment, we see their whole being, and most importantly they sense our non-judgment and support.

When we establish an environment based on trust, patients feel safe enough to be vulnerable on many levels. They confide, they are respectful and become open to recommendations. Their trust is earned over time, and it only takes one moment to break. A lapse in our healing consciousness can irrevocably change the relationship and environment for healing for patients.

To borrow from a North American Arrowhead teaching, we need to be "Aware, Awake and Alert" in each moment. Through practice, our procedures become entrained to a point of unconscious competence and we do not have to think about them. Those procedures become an automatic extension of our services. When this occurs, we are free to "sense" what is going on around us: mastering our visual observation, listening to the energy behind the words aurally, and feeling the tone of the body through palpation. We tune in with our intuition for connecting with another person.

To illustrate, I remember as a student learning to palpate and adjust. I thought I was really hallucinating in my attempts to palpate the difference between muscle, fascia, joint-play and other anatomical landmarks such as TVP's. By the time I was setting-up for an adjustment, my whole body was tense. My actions were totally in my head, mechanically thinking through each part. I was so tight there was nothing left for the adjustment, as all my muscles were already loaded.

The concept of intuitive actions applies to the performance of elite athletes. When instinctive awareness takes over, they truly become one with their activity or sport. If they become nervous, their body tenses and they lose their edge and form. Just as learning the skills of a sport, learning the mechanics and steps of Chiropractic was not easy. Through practice and experience palpating and adjusting came as second nature, without conscious thought. Akin to becoming an artist, it is difficult to breakdown and describe exactly how an adjustment is delivered: because when you think about it, you destroy it. Rather, when the adjustment is instinctive, the hands just know what to do.

When I mentor other students struggling with palpation and adjusting skills, I am reminded of what it was like for me as a student. Everyone learns differently, yet the consistency is that practice comes between performance. Learn the basics, then get out of your heads – stop thinking and begin *being*. Keep practicing, as practice leads to certainty and mastery.

Learning develops through four stages:
1. Unconscious incompetence – we do not know what we do not know.
2. Conscious incompetence – we know we do not know.
3. Conscious competence – we know what we know, but we have to think about it.
4. Unconscious Competence – we no longer have to think about it, we just do it.

Just about every learned process or set of skills goes through the stages: from learning to drive a car, to developing the skills of a trade. When daily procedures become an unconsciously competent habit, it frees our awareness to listen and observe the nuances.

This unconscious competence is core to the delivery of a masterful adjustment. The adjustment is our expression of Chiropractic. No other profession can deliver it as well as Chiropractors. The adjustment represents the cumulative integration of our Principles with our individual understanding of the anatomy, philosophy and science of the human body. It is what a patient will partly judge us by. It needs to be delivered cleanly, accurately and with focused intent. This requires confidence and certainty that is gained through repetition, observation of and critique by colleagues, and practice. There is never enough practice, as we always have potential for improving. An artist cannot say they have created their masterpiece since one to come may still be in their future. An athlete may have a personal best, but cannot know for sure they have truly turned in a *best* performance. There could always be one more, one better yet.

The Universe Gives Us What We Can Handle

At times, I may judge what has been placed before me, but know I am a co-creator in it. What I learned more than anything else is that one can be brilliant and talented, but if not lead first by the heart, it is more difficult to push ahead. I am constantly learning deeper levels of turning inwardly to ask for guidance and trust my heart and intuition, rather than my head. Whenever I have followed the advice of my head or intellect I regretted it. The conflict comes because I enjoy spending time in my head – analyzing and reflecting, debating and discussing. With recent events in my life, I am learning to let go and just be. Just being is an art. You will read about my journey in a future book yet to be published.

When faced with challenge, I realize it is a test for me to learn and grow. I may look to others who have experienced a similar event in their life. I ask how they dealt with it. Overall, the Universe will not drop more than we can handle into our lap.

People Do Not Care What You Know Until They Feel You Care

Knowing statistics and health data does not change most people's lifestyles. If it did, we would all be at our ideal weight, eating organic foods, drinking clean purified water, sleeping an appropriate amount, detoxifying, practicing mindfulness, and reducing stresses. Knowing the data does not change our behavior. Emotions, feelings and attachments change us. So in order for what we know to be heard, we need to appeal to others on their level, and meet them where they are. Once we have a relationship, eventually they become willing to hear our advice. Connect with hearts, then minds.

In making connections, I remember a particular patient, a male teenager. His dream was to become a pilot like his dad. He had severe long-term chronic asthma, and was devastated when he heard he did not qualify as a pilot due to the scarring within his lungs, and his poor pulmonary function.

In his mid-teenage years, he began being adjusted in my office on a regular basis. His use of inhalers decreased; in addition, the acute attacks that frequently sent him to the hospital Emergency wards began to reduce. I once visited him in the hospital. He was in a tent with secondary oxygen and was running a poor oxygen saturation rate. His breathing was labored, rapid, shallow, and he was using his accessory breathing muscles to assist his breathing. I asked for and was granted permission to adjust him. He was adjusted and within seconds, everything – and I mean everything – normalized. The rapid, labored breathing relaxed into rhythmic breaths, his oxygen saturation returned to within normal range, and his body relaxed. The attending nurse stood – eyes wide-open – frozen in place. Speechless. He returned home within a couple of hours.

A few years later, I received a thank you note from his mother stating her sons' dream to become a pilot became reality. He had no lung scarring and pulmonary function tests were within qualifying ranges. He had no medication and no bouts of asthma.

We connect with people and help them to connect with their dreams. We make a difference in people's lives. These experiences allow us to gain a quiet certainty with what we do. A confidence in knowing that no matter what is going on from the outside in, if the inside is not communicating, then the rest does not matter. The presence of life allows the body to be organized. Interference with life reduces efficiency of the body's ability to function properly. If the body cannot perceive its environment accurately and resend at its full magnitude, then it will respond with a less than favorable adaptive choice, perhaps making an error in the process by finding a less than ideal way. If the body continues to operate this way over time it deteriorates human vitality.

Who We Unfold To Become

We all experience rough times and bumpy roads along our path, as they are a part of life. It's not the obstacles that are most important, but rather who we become as a result of overcoming them. As an example, in a span of a few years a number of personal challenges were thrown my way. In respect for time, I explain with minimal detail by saying there were the unrelated deaths of my godmother, my father-in-law, my father, my sister-in-law and our oldest sixteen-year-old dog. In the same year, I had another dog hit and dragged by a truck and survive, a mother who had congestive heart failure, a mother-in-law who suffered an extensive stroke, and a brother who's experimental brain surgery kept him in the ICU for twelve weeks during the SARS epidemic. In addition, I had a vehicular accident, when my car skidded on black ice, rolled-over and crossed two lanes of on-coming traffic. With all of these events I did not slow down, but kept my usual pace. These significant events were not fully dealt with; I just chalked them up as more life experience. I dealt with them intellectually, but not emotionally. I shifted more into my head and stayed there. I kept myself busy, which was the first clue I was not fully connecting with my feelings.

Dealing with my emotions was inconvenient. I did not want to stop what I was doing. My avoidance was excused by not having time to feel. Over time, life slowly began to feel more difficult and I became frustrated with any little mishap. Being strong, I muscled through it all using my stamina and endurance, focusing on the tasks needing to be completed. I was so busy *doing* I did not see it.

I recognized my disconnection when I finally caught myself saying, "I think;" whereas I more commonly say, "I feel." A variety of other events also occurred to the point I had to literally stop to reassess who I was and how I defined myself. The *doing* stopped so I could just focus on *being*. Over the years, my neurology has been wired to the process of *activity* and *busy-ness*, and to stop long enough to change my neurology felt cruelly difficult.

"There is no process which does not require time," Principle #6 of Stephenson's 33 Principles. Knowing this still becomes difficult to apply. For someone accustomed to being busy, allowing time to unravel is not an easy transition for change. A principle in neuroscience is: "Neurons that Fire together, Wire together." The reverse is also true. So I worked on reversing my neurological wiring.

With my re-evaluation of who I was unfolding to become, I began loving the down time. I needed to be reminded of *who* I am and distinguish it from *what* I do. In retrospect, it was quite plain that my outer world was reflecting my inner world. I am thankful to the Universe for providing me with the chaotic challenges, for they served as a wake up call to making change.

'Response – Ability' is aptly named because humans live and experience life through their nervous system. Our ability to respond has everything to do with the quality and quantity of our nervous system function. A healthy response is free to be creative. Through our 'response – ability' we communicate who we are to the world. In our practices, our ability to palpate demonstrates and communicates to patients our wisdom supporting what we do. In life, our response to the world determines outcomes. What we are capable of 'seeing and not seeing' is dictated by the limitations in our perception and experience. Our ability to adapt in the world determines our survival and health. Responsibility is an inside out process.

When we adjust our thoughts and adjust our actions, we adjust our life. Like Chiropractic, when life is *pure* it is without a doubt *powerful.*

> It is not the strongest of the species that survives. It is not the fastest of the species that survives. It is the one most able to adapt to change.
> ~ *Charles Darwin*

- To help others, first change yourself.
- There is no failure, only lessons.
- Ask for help and it appears.
- Continue being a student of life.
- Love them when they do not love themselves.
- We each have a unique path – celebrate it!
- The journey is everything.

Living And Leading A Vital Life
Dr. Janice Hughes

I no longer have the privilege every day of adjusting people. My own search for vitalism and living a life of vitality is the reason this occurred.

I now realize the messages about vitalism I've received along my path were delivered to teach and encourage me to stand up and be *me*. I'm a strong and driven woman, in roles and positions in my profession that – to date – have not had many women involved. In challenging the *status quo* and trying new things, I began to create opportunities to truly define vitalism for myself. My path is to get the message out to other women that you can be more. By embracing vitalism, you can be incredibly powerful.

Vitalism in action has shown me:
- ♦ Balance is an illusion, but being in the flow is not.
- ♦ We can succeed in spite of ourselves.
- ♦ Discipline determines our destiny.
- ♦ Wisdom is recognizing that any adversity has incredible benefits.
- ♦ Life is all vibration, at a deep cellular level, and expressing our unique vibration creates a life of authenticity.
- ♦ Life is good!

What Is Vitalism?

Vitalism is the doctrine that life involves immaterial and incorporeal 'vital forces,' and cannot be explained scientifically. This subtle essence is what we – as Chiropractors – come close to touching every day with every adjustment. Vitalism is not unique and specific to Chiropractic. Chiropractors did not create this word and its use is certainly not exclusive to us. Although, because it is such a critical part of practicing Chiropractic, it is one of our guiding Principles.

The challenge for so many of us in the profession is that some days we forget about this magic and connection to vitalism. We get caught in the business reality of running a practice, raising a family, or daily to-do lists. Yet, all it takes is adjusting an infant and seeing almost instant changes to remind us that we have influence on that subtle substance, that vital life force within people.

More than ever before, there is currently a focus on what is vitalistic versus mechanistic. Philosophically, mechanism is the theory that Laws of Nature can explain all natural phenomena. In opposition, vitalism postulates that organisms have 'vital forces' that are not physical. In our current day there is greater awareness of the concept of vitalism as it pertains to health care, food, and life in general.

In the world of a healer, vitalism is expressed and revealed to each of us in unique ways. There are so many phenomenal women writing in this book about their lives and connection to vitalism. Since many of them are currently still in practice, I know and trust they will be sharing healing examples of vitalism truly at play. For this reason I chose to focus on the consistent vitalism in my life. Vitalism was distinctly full force in my practice, yet in hindsight I have come to realize how it was vitalism at work in my life that has created my entire path in life.

Three *Acts* Of Life

Several years ago I read an amazing interview with Jane Fonda speaking about the stages of her life, similar to acts in a play. She referenced three distinct acts, and in looking back saw a thread of connection. She said while living through those days, it felt like three distinct and separate lives, with a different focus in each. This is so similar to a stage play, where often the second act is so distinctly different than the first act. The third act is often where all the details and pieces from the earlier acts are linked and connected.

At this point in my own life – what I would call the middle of my second act – I can honor and see the role vitalism has played in every aspect. Vitalism attracted me to Chiropractic, basically before I really even knew anything about it. It was just a sense I had as I first experienced Chiropractic myself. Without knowing anything about Chiropractic school or education, I applied based on the experience of my own first adjustments.

I had traveled a much more traditional educational route. My first degree was in Microbiology at a university where I thought I would likely apply to Veterinarian school. Really having no idea what I truly wanted to pursue, I then moved on to another university for a post-graduate degree, specializing in Somatic Cell Genetics. Obviously this was moving me closer in the direction of traditional medicine, particularly choosing a university with a phenomenal medical school.

During my years in university, I was really focused on the pursuit of knowledge. I can't say I was choosing things consciously, or really thinking about the influence my choices would have on the rest of my life. The unique part of my education was my involvement with research of eukaryotic cells, and the impact of various environmental stimuli on their growth rates. The overall research was in the area of cancer research, and if anything, I was really learning more what I didn't want to do with the rest of my life.

My research work was almost too many years ago now to count. Yet even at that time, some very bright minds in this field were already aware that the genetic make up of a cell is inducible. This means that you aren't only a product of your DNA, as several environmental parameters and factors impact DNA synthesis. Little did I realize this essentially addresses Vitalism!

All of the reading and reference work I was required to do (thanks to a very meticulous and excellent advisor, although I didn't always think so at the time) was also teaching me a lot about research design. This background distinctly influences my learning to this day. I realize so many articles and much of research are based on a design to make the numbers represent or illustrate what we want them to show. I also learned to cross through conventional subject and topic lines. There are often papers, research, and insights from a totally different field playing a large role in the work of a researcher. Rather than sticking to an assigned discipline, being creative with the approach of research sparks flares of genius.

Throughout my research experience I was truly more fascinated with the really creative personalities of the researchers and people I met than the actual work. Realizing I didn't want to be a researcher, yet so far down the traditional medical path, I felt a bit trapped.

With my infinite wisdom at the time, I decided to take some time off to travel; in other words, ran away. I had no illusion that I would find myself, or my answers, in travel. I just knew I needed a break. Backpacking in Europe didn't strike me with insight; yet I *do* know that stepping away was a critical piece in being open to change for moving forward.

Months later I was back in the same routine. Interestingly, within weeks of being back, I was injured. All of my traditional medical connections and buddies were talking about bed rest and the long- term repercussions of my injury.

I called my dad, who had been seeing a Chiropractor for many years. I went to visit his Chiropractor, and within three adjustments I was 70-75 percent improved. Now it wasn't so much the improvement that made me stop in my tracks. It was that casually the Chiropractor mentioned that with all my school and training I'd make a great Chiropractor. "Hhhmmmm."

The Act Of Becoming A Chiropractor

It was as if the seed was planted. Knowing very little about Chiropractic, my investigation told me there was one college in Canada at that time. I discovered I was within the deadline of applying for the following September, and began to complete my application. I reinvested in my research with a new zeal and target: I needed to be done so I could head to Chiropractic school. Now remember, this was all basically without knowing much at all about this *thing* called Chiropractic. It just gave me a newfound target and direction.

Little did I know, it was very difficult to be accepted into this one school in Canada, Canadian Memorial Chiropractic College (CMCC). I was granted an interview, and my interview was basically welcoming me to the college. Only upon starting that fall did I realize I was 'accepted' because of my multiple degrees. This was a phase and time in Chiropractic when it very much focused on validity and credibility within the medical profession. There were several of us in my class with post-graduate degrees. Because of my advanced degree, I was exempt from a number of the early courses in the curriculum.

Entering into Chiropractic school was a whirlwind beginning with the completion of my Masters Degree, dealing with the critical comments about leaving, and dealing with family wondering what I would do with yet another degree and asking when 'enough was enough;' all this strife for just trusting a feeling. It was almost like listening to the whispers in the wind. Not having a logical reason or seeing the full picture and vision, I still trusted. Many would say my pursuit was stubbornness, and with my strong personality that would have been a fair comment.

The act of trusting and pursuing enabled me to quickly connect with sincerely vital and unique characters. Several were classmates from many parts of the country. Steven Silk, Greg Woolfrey, and Margaret were three individuals that were more vital and free spirited than one could imagine! These three impacted my entire first year, and were instrumental in showing me success comes in many forms and ways. One such 'full of life' instructor, Dr. Keith Innes, was involved in our anatomy lab. He challenged many of us to search outside of the traditional schooling for success Principles and growth. He created opportunities for many students at CMCC to train in Gonstead and Motion Palpation at his clinic, and learn skills and expand our horizons.

Dr. Keith also created an opportunity for me to work at his clinic during the summer, and again part-time throughout my Chiropractic training. The skill sets I learned in billing, report writing, front desk client management, and many other clinical procedures are all attributed to working within a really vital and active clinic.

Along my path in Chiropractic college I was able to search for and follow greatness. Being exempt from some basic science classes gave me extra time other students did not have. I used my extra time well, following around senior interns in clinic, visiting successful Chiropractors, and learning from truly wonderful and successful role models. Success and greatness leave clues!

My path in education taught me learning comes in many forms. I learned more outside the traditional classroom. To this day I continue to consider this critical. Our schools are entrusted to educate students formally, and ensure the passing of board exams. With the regulating boards accrediting institutions requiring a certain number of credits for specific course curriculum, there is just not enough hours in the day to teach all the success Principles and key points for creating successful practices and lives. A lot of this responsibility is on the shoulders of graduates. It behooves each of us in the profession to find better ways to support and balance learning both inside the system and outside the system.

The Vital Act Of Becoming A Mother

Now obviously I didn't have enough on my plate. During school I began living with my husband and life partner, David Boynton. Part way through my third year of school and during Dave's first year of practice we became pregnant. I think this time in my life taught me more about vitality and the capacity of each of us than any other time, juggling clinic, X-ray Rotations, and pregnancy. CMCC had traditional academic years, and internship between third and fourth year during the summer. I realized that summer as an intern was my opportunity to 'practice' and treat Clinic like a real practice. My due date was at the beginning of the fourth year, and I set my goals to be finished with my clinic requirements even before I delivered. This way I could focus on the new baby and classes, without the pressures of clinic requirements.

Of course there are plans, and then there is real life! Yes, I finished clinic requirements. However, then it was time to keep client/patient care going, deliver a baby, and be back at classes and X-ray Rotations within ten days of having the baby. Throughout this blur was the magical experience of having a child, and making vitalistic choices of natural child birth, choosing not to vaccinate based on my microbiology education, and watching and learning the power of the adjustment.

My son Rob became the first child that many in my class checked and adjusted. Thanks to so many in my class, who juggled Rob in the intern's room and hallways, I was able to finish requirements and expectations. Rob was also such a natural lesson to so many of us of the power of the adjustment, and its significance in smoothly moving a child through the early months of life.

My last year of Chiropractic school was also a whirlwind. Within this year I had a baby, finished classes, got married, wrote board exams, and was ready to launch into the real world of practice. What the heck did that mean? I hadn't even had a chance to catch my breath, let alone decide what I wanted to do. The one guiding Principle was that on some level I realized I didn't know what I didn't know.

Now the good news is that the one thing I *did* know was for Dave and I we could either have a practice together, or a marriage. Both would not mix! We are simply very different and distinct personalities. Many people we know, and I have since coached, can manage the collaboration of both roles. Luckily Dave and I knew and honored that this was not the case for us.

By 'coincidence' a favorable circumstance presented for me to cover a practice many miles away from where Dave was practicing. An amazing Chiropractor with a long and established practice and legacy had broken his wrist. The position was there for me to cover his practice for 4-6 weeks. Dave stepped-in and created the opportunity for me to leave and cover this practice, and gain incredible experience on the adjusting front. This opportunity enhanced my skills and most importantly my confidence.

Practice Reveals Life Lessons

During my time as a cover Doctor, two Chiropractic friends approached me with an invitation to join their growing and thriving practice. They were looking for an associate. Why not? Without another plan of where I wanted to live or what type of practice I wanted to establish, this was an opportunity with great people. Of course the driving distance and crazy hours never entered my thoughts.

I started in the most non-traditional format. Practicing hours that in hindsight are not ideal for building *any* type of practice. Yet I didn't know at the time. As I mentioned, I didn't know what I didn't know. I just knew I was destined for success, and that I loved this thing called Chiropractic. With vital energy as my fire I set out to accomplish what I knew at a core level.

Fortunate for me, within my first few months of practice the Doctors I practiced with, Steve and Annette, took me to a life-altering seminar. I spent a weekend with Dr. John Demartini and a group of highly successful Doctors and human beings. I look back now, and even then on some level realized it was a life changing experience for me. The seminar offered tangible knowledge and experience to a level of knowingness about Universal Principles and life at a deep and core level.

Dr. John, with his messages and knowledge, became my strongest mentor. The coaching and success Principles I was guided to with his mentorship launched my success to establish congruent and consistent actions to create a phenomenal practice.

Anyone that has heard me speak from stage knows I talk a lot about my blunders and challenges along the way. They are a part of life and a part of practice. I have probably done and said more things wrong than you could ever imagine. The distinction is that I was constantly in action. I was setting goals and targets, and appropriate action steps to create those goals. I was incredibly disciplined. Discipline determines your destiny!

Vital can be defined simply as being full of life, full of spirit. My connection to the vitalistic Principles of Chiropractic, as well as my passion for life and sharing the Chiropractic message blended to create a magnetic energy within my practice and life. I was succeeding in spite of myself.

Dr. John also taught me to think globally. Instead of just focusing on my practice, I thought how I could serve my community, the Chiropractic profession in my country, as well as Chiropractic worldwide. I hung an enormous poster of the World in my office, covering the entire wall, and began sticking pins in place of where people came from to be adjusted in my office. Obviously it started with a small number of pins. Yet, is it any 'coincidence' that suddenly people visiting family from Russia, Yugoslavia, and many other places in the world were suddenly on my clinic doorstep?

During this early stage of my career I stepped up and became involved in the political association for Chiropractors in my local area. The Universal Principles were also teaching me to have a voice in decisions that impact my ability to practice in the fashion I love. As I have mentioned, this was a stage in Chiropractic that held acceptance foremost in reverence. It was important to me, and I was passionate about honoring what was unique and distinct about Chiropractic. I left the traditional system, and became so involved in Chiropractic because of vitalism and the unique ability to address it within our scope of practice. Having a voice, and representing wellness and vitalism in the profession was critical to me.

Another vital element to my plan was to attract and groom a vital team. I knew I needed support in the clinic, and to have a well-trained team. It became imperative for me to introduce the members of my team to people and places of learning in Chiropractic. We travelled to seminars to enhance our knowledge, and rejuvenate our inspiration. Sharing these same Principles of life and Chiropractic with my first Chiropractic Assistant, Rhonda was critical in fine tuning her procedures, as well as shaping and developing our capacity within the clinic. Interesting is the large number of people we could serve, just one CA and I. We were fortunate to become connected with Dr. Guy Riekeman and his Quest seminar system. His seminar was instrumental in assisting us in developing the systems and the support team to be able to serve and help even more people.

Throughout the first five years of my practice, I was so fortunate to be around great people that shared with me incredible Principles, methods, procedures and more.

Ask and you shall receive. On several occasions, I *quieted* my mind through meditation and prayer, and asked for guidance. Without delay, the next teacher or opportunity presented. One such example is Dr. Peter Amlinger handing me my first copies of the *Green Books*. I'd obviously lived in a shell until then, because I didn't' know such recorded writings existed! He handed me two books at a political meeting, and now I simply smile at the juxtaposition of 'philosophical' writings handed to me at a political meeting.

It's so important for me to thank and honor each person that came into my life along this early path of my career. I realize my success has been totally related to the quality of the people around me, and the books that I've read. And most of those books were presented or shared with me by the people around me, an example of vitalism in action.

The patients in this early phase of my career taught me more than I could ever even possibly put into words. When I opened up to the *bigness* of Chiropractic, and when anyone does, the floodgates are lifted. I was presented with cases and examples of every type of condition and disorder. The more I focused on the uniqueness of Chiropractic, and on being a nervous system specialist, the more the results spoke for themselves. The vitalistic Principles at work created even more passion and commitment for me to helping more and more people.

Stepping Into Uniqueness

I was so fortunate to share this path and time in life with my husband Dave. Vitality is truly put to the test when you run a large and growing practice, and also then try to figure out how to juggle and run a full and vital family. Without my husband Dave I'm not sure this would have been feasible. Dave and my son Rob played such a vital role in supporting my growth as a person. The same Universal Principles that applied to my practice, applied to my life. The discipline to create the time and present-time focus and consciousness on my family life was critical.

The ability to create flow in life and practice for many women in Chiropractic presents challenges distinct to females. There are physical differences between men and women in practice, yet I feel those pale in comparison to the psychological and relationship differences. It's not like one path is easier than another, just different and unique. I found myself in territory that was different from even the women around me. Some of the women Chiropractors I knew, and women in various business models, were focusing more on family while their children were younger. Practicing part time or staying home with my sons just simply didn't fit my personality style.

I had my middle and youngest sons while I was practicing full time in a large and vital practice. At this point in my career, I had not yet addressed an associate based practice model. The buck stopped with me. There were some interesting times and challenges in making decisions on how to manage the practice while pregnant, and more importantly manage my time out of the office once the babies were born.

As anyone reading this might realize, not everyone in our profession focuses on vitalism. When creating a vital, and on some days crazy, style of practice, not many people can simply cover that type of office. Many people that visited or heard about my office would profess to want this type of model. Yet in reality there were very few people willing to do the things that it takes to create it, on both the physical and mental level.

Fortunate for me, trust and faith in a bigger picture allowed me to attract great-fitting cover doctors for my practice. And no coincidence, one doctor who covered my practice is a contributing author to this book! Having coverage for my maternity leaves was obviously critical. Yet it took the right people to be able to keep my crazy practice alive and well.

On a deep level I find women doctors have the capacity to touch and connect with the vitalistic life force within others. The women doctors that covered for me, as well as the many female students I have work with, mentored or coached have all shown me their intuitive and creative ability to grasp the essence of vitalism. No coincidence that one online dictionary site describes an example of vitalism as *"a dynamic full of life woman."* Within each woman, there is a unique blend of empathy, intuition, love and caring.

Going from one child to three over a short period of time can only be described as a team on a sports field going from man-to-man coverage to zone coverage. My husband Dave and I were quickly out-numbered. Welcome to a new level of life and craziness at our household. My personal winning strategy during my pregnancy with my middle son Jackson was to hire a professional coach. Coaching Principles, along with the systems of education I learned through Dr. Riekeman and his mentoring were instrumental in shifting my practice into a stronger business model.

After my youngest son, Kobi, was born, my coach helped me to streamline my office hours and systems, and assisted me in becoming open to the help and support I needed for success in the office and at home. Becoming a stronger leader in my office, versus just doing all of the work, was imperative. Planning and organizing at home was even more essential. Coaching enabled me to pull out of myself the model and systems that felt authentic to me, and that created an even deeper expression of vitalism in my life and practice.

What Next?

Facilitated by coaches in my life asking me deeper and more inner driven questions, the time came for me to open up to my dreams and aspirations for the future. In some ways I was already living my purpose, based on the purpose and vision statements I created within the first year of my practice. "What is next?" The question kept running through my mind.

When we begin to ask questions, it is really a signal for a transitional phase in our life and career. Luckily for me, with great coaching and mentorship, I didn't just jump or run into the next pursuit and/or project. Hastiness can be a trap. I had great guidance with building-in personal time and dreamtime. I began tapping into the 'what is next.'

While our younger two boys were little, I made the decision not to travel as much to seminars, or to remain as heavily involved with politics. Instead, I didn't want to be doing things that were not high on my list of values. In learning to prioritize, I realized some elements within the roles I took-on had become tolerations. It was necessary for me to recognize it was of my own doing. My longing to be involved and have a voice had filled my plate entirely. It was okay to learn to give myself permission to step back, and focus completely on the top priorities in my life.

Prioritizing served as valuable instruction for me to listen to my inner voice, and act in accordance with my own inner values. My destiny wasn't about what other people said or thought. I'd created these roles, and it would have been easier to keep doing them (particularly at the level I had begun to be involved in the politics and some other aspects of my career) than to step down. Yet it was time to learn to find the language to explain, and switch my focus and direct my energy to the areas that truly mattered the most to me. Then muster the courage to do it!

The more I learned about powerful decision making tools and living one's best life, the more I wanted to learn and grow in ways to help my patients or others utilize these same tools. Because of the flexibility of training available to become a personal and professional coach, it was an avenue that could continue to fuel my thirst for knowledge, learning and growing. This is inherent in a lot of us, and can become the trap of why we keep thinking we need to be on the seminar circuit, or always learning new things. Seminars are powerful when we indeed tap into the pure growth aspect of them, but I realized I didn't have to tie it directly to my current profession. Here was another lesson for me in crossing disciplines.

Again, hindsight is 20-20. I realize my training as a coach was enabling me to put language and tools into place to work with people at a deep level of thoughts and beliefs. I began to apply my newly learned language and tools to asking my patients strong and powerful questions. I asked them questions about what was blocking their vital flow or creating physical/health challenge within their lives. Designing workshops and seminars for my patients and local community, all around coaching principles, helped me step into my next role of coaching and guiding people.

Each step of the way I was fortunate to be continually guided by skilled and talented coaches and mentors. Several of these mentors began to ask me to speak and teach more within the Chiropractic profession. The more this happened, the more my 'next step' in the journey was revealed. I developed the vitality and love of speaking to accompany my new role. The more I embraced the journey, and continued to do things that brought love and joy into my life, the more the other details and pieces fell into place to allow me to follow my purposeful path. Within the practice, my associate, Dr. Shaelyn Osborn, was ready, willing and able to step-up to take on a role of leadership and ownership of the clinic. I had the support of my family, as well as my family of patients.

The most difficult phase of my journey was departing from hands-on healing. Adjusting and connecting with others at their core level came natural and was innate to me. Once I was able to connect with a very deep level of myself, coaching and leading others in our profession truly enabled me to touch everyone and everything in their lives, including *their* patients! Becoming a coach enabled me to focus my intention and skills towards seeing greatness in other Chiropractors. There are many days where I see more in others than they are able to see in themselves. Revealing their inner wisdom for them to embrace creates passion and enthusiasm within me, and keeps fueling my vital flame.

Skills For Moving Into My Next Act

Another aspect of vitalism in my life (and probably the most significant) was becoming a charismatic leader. The process first started with me focusing on leading myself – my internal world and my life. Then, I began expressing my inner clarity to the outer world. Based on my core value of *authenticity*, the expression of my 'insides' on the 'outside' was extremely important. In the family model my husband Dave and I designed, the same theme flowed naturally with parenting our children. We wanted to lead and inspire our children towards greatness, and encourage their expression of their true selves to the world. In Chiropractic, my role and path is to inspire the next generation of Chiropractic leaders.

To date, my connection to my values has been one of the most essential elements in the plan for my life. My values have connected me to my guiding Principles. These have a flair and flavor very similar to the guiding Principles of Chiropractic. Without guiding Principles we can waiver on even basic daily decisions. *With* guiding Principles, decisions and directions are inherently natural, and you create a life path that feels uniquely authentic.

I still don't completely know what the next *Act* is for me. I do know it is essential to make-way for flow (vitalism in action). Honoring the flow of intelligence by listening and trusting our intuition enables us to express innate through the body and throughout our entire lives. Experiences that bring joy and passion increase this flow. Things that feel heavy and uninspiring decrease our vibration and block the natural flow. By blending *right* feelings, with *right* actions, based on *right* values equals an inspired and vital life. By promoting flow in my life, I have been fortunate to create the opportunity to work with Dr. Joan Fallon and her biotechnology company, *Curemark*. Joan's established company and her work with Autism (and other unmet neurological needs) are completely based on a set of values and Principles not only she aligns with, but I align with also. Every day I love what I do, and continue learning an incredible amount. I watch as Joan sets up her company in a unique and inspired way. I call it a 'soulful' company, based on values and high standards. And every day we break new ground.

In some ways, I feel each day creates more clarity for me, enabling me to see the thread of connections throughout all of the various things I have done and been involved with in my life. In following the flow and path, I am happier and more satisfied than I ever imagined. Every new lesson reminds me to trust and honor the vitalistic life force within – rather than fighting and controlling, just allow the flow. I listen to the *whispers in the wind*.

A Vital Life

Vitalism, to me, is so natural and authentic.

I don't want to leave the impression that living a vital life is easy. None of my own paths has been or *felt* easy. Yet basing the pieces of my life on the core Principle of vitalism has carried me along a successful journey. Vitalism can be felt and identified – it's a vibration, an aura, a mojo that people may exude. You might label it as passion, or even enthusiasm, but to me it is vitalism. Did you know the word "enthusiasm" comes from the two little Greek words *en* and *theos*? Enthusiasm literally means *"God within."* How cool is that? The outward expression of an inner vitalism can literally be a connection to the God within each of us.

My wish is that you may find *your* path, *your* authentic life. In sharing my own, I hope to spark *your* inner greatness.

As my dear friend Dr. Fred Barge would have said, "*Enuf* said!"

- **Stand up and celebrate your uniqueness.**
- **Balance is an illusion but being in the flow is not.**
- **We can succeed in spite of ourselves.**
- **Do less to be more.**
- **Life is all vibration, at a deep cellular level, and expressing our unique vibration creates a life of authenticity.**
- **Life is good!**

It Is Not Just One Thing
Dr. Cecile Thackeray

Health exists when the normally constructed body properly performs its functions. Disease is a condition in which the organs or organism is abnormally related to internal or external influences, which relates to our welfare physically, mentally or spiritually. Disease is, therefore, a general term signifying any variation from the normal either in functions or tissue or both. An alteration of function cannot occur without a corresponding change in the structure of the tissue. It is possible, however, that the structural change in the functionary organ may be so slight as to remain undetected by the most precise method of differential diagnosis known by pathological investigators.
~ *D.D. Palmer*

I didn't grow up wanting to be a Chiropractor; instead I wanted to be a pediatric neurosurgeon. Intuitively I knew I never wanted to stand in front of anyone telling them their child did not make it through the surgery. However, I was fascinated by the intricacies of the brain and the ability of it to control and coordinate the billions of functions and actions. How does it work? It was magical, powerful and had an essence all of its own. BUT, what happened when things went wrong? What happened when that communication was broken?

Lucky for me I was being lead in a different professional direction, and was fortunate enough to have experienced and witnessed some great things through Chiropractic. As a matter of fact, it changed my life – although I didn't know it at the time.

I fell off of a bunk bed at the age of two and proceeded to develop allergies, and osteomyelitis (bacterial infection of the bone marrow) after falling off my bike. Then, at the onset of puberty I started to suffer from serious migraines and could not function for several days at a time. Well, I didn't appear to have any *serious* ramifications in the eyes of the doctors, so I must have been okay, or so they said. What was happening to my immune system? My nervous system? And my ability to adapt to stress or foreign activity?

I remember as a young child lying awake at night thinking – this just can't be right! Who would want to live like this? Thankfully my mother was an open-minded woman and listened to a friend of ours who worked for a Chiropractor. Her friend said a few other patients with headaches had great relief and suggested we give it a try.

I went to be adjusted and within a couple of months the migraines were diminishing both in frequency and intensity. I remember thinking how wonderful it was to have a change in symptoms without any medications, even when told by other doctors I would grow out of needing them.

In the case of my mother, she suffered for years with chronic lower back issues due to a compression injury. With this, she gave birth spontaneously at seven months gestation to her third child, a premature son (my brother). My mother had an emergency hysterectomy following his birth, and he spent most of his first year of life in the hospital with a re-occurring collapsed lung. A fluke, a coincidence? I think not!

My mother wore a back brace for many years following her injury and surgery until she tried Chiropractic. Could her injury have disempowered her nervous system function?

I look back in my life and wonder about these things. When I was in the fourth grade, a very close family friend's son died of leukemia at the age of six. Apart from being so sad watching their family suffer, I remember again wondering what causes the body to become diseased? Why do some people just stop adapting and *WHY* can't they overcome it? Does the attack of a foreign substance cause the body to have a complete melt down? Did something happen to this child when he was given his shots? Did he have trauma at birth? He wasn't born that way! Why at the age of two? *WHY-WHY-WHY?* I cried myself to sleep feeling pain for his family, for our family, but mostly for him.

This boy was a very spiritual being; he knew things most people his age would never understand or know. He understood love; he understood relationships; and he understood pain. He knew he was put on earth to teach people to experience love, even for a brief moment, and to let go of our fears of living. I remember standing in the schoolyard when he went into the hospital for the last time. I stood thinking that it was now time to grow up. I had to be smart and I had to make something of myself. I felt his death wasn't fair and it fueled me with desire to figure out why things like this occur.

Well, I still haven't figured it out. But I do know these events in my life instilled a passion deep within me – a passion so strong, I don't even fully comprehend it. These events put me on the quest to not only understand the human body, but the human mind and the relationship of the two. *Why* has been one of my favorite questions.

I can't say for sure if just one thing made me want to become a Chiropractor, but I am certain I was being strongly pulled in its direction. For these reasons as well as many others along the way, I continue to be a very passionate Chiropractor. Admittedly, I sometimes lose my way, but always seem to be thrown back in the direction of vitalistic energy and purity. I know Chiropractic can't help everything, but it certainly can't hurt to try!

As a base, let's recall Chiropractic Principle #4, *The Triune of Life* – "Life is a triunity having three necessary united factors, namely, Intelligence, Force and Matter." I used to think Chiropractors could save the world, and the hardest lesson for me to learn was Chiropractic Principle #24, *The Limits of Adaptation* – "Innate Intelligence adapts forces and matter for the body as long as it can do so without breaking a Universal Law, or is limited by the limitations of matter." I always wanted to believe that if the forces of intelligence were present, the matter could always improve. Instead, I realize I have to accept there *are* limits.

However, removing interferences in the body to relieve the nerve interference is paramount for proper function – no matter what. With this understanding in mind, the most amazing things have come before my eyes, most certainly because of my confidence in adjusting children and babies. My thanks and appreciation to Larry Webster my mentor – God rest his soul. Also, I *know* I had guidance from my little friend in heaven.

Changing One Life At A Time

An eighteen-month old child had not yet in his life slept through a night. A healthy sleep pattern for this age is about eleven hours of solid sleep at night, with two or three hours of napping during the days. He was sick about 80 percent of the time with colds, congestion and earaches. No one could figure out why he was always sick. Supposedly his birth was normal, though I was not there to witness it. He was nursed until the age of fourteen months. His family had a fairly good understanding of nutrition and made several different attempts to correct his issues with a modified diet. They didn't want to use another course of antibiotics, because it did not resolve the problem.

Not by any means were they strung at their last hope, but the mother was literally exhausted and didn't know where else to turn. Thus far, everything they had tried did not improve her infant's condition. Alas, they were referred to our office by one of her close friends.

I remember seeing this child and thinking what a miserable existence he must have been enduring. He could not communicate what was wrong, could not begin to know how to fix it or how to even help himself in anyway. During his examination, I felt an incredible stress inside. Most likely because I placed myself in the shoes of his mother, wondering how she managed seeing him in his condition – and I had only been with him for forty-five minutes.

In the examination most everything appeared normal, *except* for a distended stomach, discomfort upon palpation of the lower left abdominal quadrant, and a diminished pupillary response reflex. Then, when I palpated the boys' cervical spine, the lateral mass of C1 was extremely prominent to the left. I had never felt anything like it before in my life! It was *palpable*, and stuck out so far it felt like you could hang a hat on it. I will never forget the feeling – so unreal it made me nauseous. Without saying a word, I rechecked his pupillary responses, as I thought, "This poor child!"

I had adjusted children and newborns before, but I knew something was seriously wrong with this baby. I knew I needed to pull myself together in order to adjust this child. I excused myself from the exam room, went into my office and looked at my very favorite picture on pages 171 and 172 of the book *The Subluxation Specific – The Adjustment Specific* (Palmer). This picture served two purposes for me. One, to remind me of the devastating effects of subluxation; and two, to give me the guidance in adjusting this child to remove the nerve interference from his brainstem.

While my assistant held the boy, I escorted the parents to the report room to present a few charts explaining what I found to be going on with their son. I then proceeded to explain what I was going to do in light of the findings. I remember telling them, as far as I was concerned, the amount of stress being caused by this one vertebra was extremely overwhelming for their son, but I didn't have any idea if removing it would help his condition. They were willing to give it a try; in fact, they were all for it.

We returned to the examination room, where he was fussing in the arms of my assistant. I was able to calm the child as taught by my mentor. I set up to adjust him, delivered one specific adjustment to correct the lateral atlas and left everything else alone. I told them he needed to be checked again the next day, and they went home.

That evening, I tried to reach the family to ask how everyone was doing. No answer, I was only able to reach their answering machine. I remember struggling through the night, hoping and praying he was okay with the adjustment. I would be lying if I didn't admit I had concern with my own abilities as a Chiropractor. I settled my thoughts by imagining what my mentor would have done. Although this was not a devastating life or death situation, I think the severity of the subluxation caused me to question my abilities and the power of the body to heal.

The next morning, I was at my practice adjusting by 6:30 AM; they were scheduled to come in at 9:00 AM. However, they did not show! Our office procedure was to make calls about fifteen minutes after a missed appointment, but at 9:40 AM my staff came to me, pulling me aside to ask what they should do. Oddly enough, my staff did not want to call because they thought everyone might be sleeping. I suggested they wait and call around noon, crossing my fingers hoping they were right.

Just after 11:00 AM we received a phone call from the family apologizing for missing the appointment, and hoping to reschedule.

So, at noon they all walked in: mother, baby, along with Grandmother and Grandfather! Mom sat down in the consultation area, and when I walked in she lit up with the biggest smile on her face. She introduced me to her parents who just stared at me.

"What did you do to my child?" She said in excitement. "My son slept for twelve hours last night; and so I did! I think I just passed out. I ran into his bedroom this morning wondering if he was still alive. My husband must have snuck out of the house this morning, as he certainly didn't want to wake either of us." She went on explaining, "My son is a completely different child today. He had a nap yesterday afternoon as soon as we put him in the car seat after leaving your office. He was awake for about three hours, and then went to bed around 9:30 PM and slept right through the night – for the first time ever! We are so grateful to you!"

Of course when a patient speaks like this to you, the ego wants to take over and say, "You are welcome." However, it is arrested by the words of the late Dr. Fred Barge, "Take no credit – Take no blame."

That day, I felt in my heart my purpose was greater than I had even realized, and I would not have to look for guidance from anything other than my own skills and intuition. I still wanted to run and read more research. I wanted to find the real reasons, to know why this was not written in the literature. I wanted to know why this happened; and most importantly, I wanted to learn more about the brain, the nervous system, and the effects of subluxation on the body.

Another one of my patients asked me if I could look at her grandchild, as he had a big lump on the side of his head. "The nurses said he did not really suffered any birth trauma because he was born via caesarean section."

"I'm happy to check him out." Inviting her to bring him to the office.

She asked, "Would a movie of his birth help you at all?"

I was excited she asked, as I had recently attended the International Pediatric Conference in Boston. At the conference, we watched several films and viewed many pictures of the birthing process, though none of anyone I knew personally.

The next day, the grandmother came in with a copy of the video, and booked an appointment for her grandchild the following day. Upon reviewing the video, I was shocked to see the child was handled like a wheel barrel whose wheel (head) was stuck in the mud. The delivery team held firmly on the handles (legs), trying to free the wheel. In order to bring this child out of the womb, they were twisting and turning the legs back and forth. Even though at seminars and through my studies I have seen videos and pictures, when I watched this particular one I just about threw-up. The baby was truly stuck, and this was their only solution for saving his life.

I thought, "What kind of damage could this cause? Could this have caused an intracranial bleed?"

The little six-week old child came into the office in the afternoon. There was a large hematoma (multi-colored, purple, blue and reddish) about the size of the babies fist. It protruded from the back of the head over to the left side just above the occiput. As the baby grew it wasn't getting any smaller. In fact, the mother thought it may be even a little larger, but confirmed it had not decreased in size since it developed shortly after birth.

The mother looked at me and asked, "Do you think you can help?"

Well, I wasn't really sure and I told her so, and also said, "I will examine him for nervous system interference in his body and let you know of my findings."

Sure enough, on the left side of his six-week young little neck he had two areas of segmental dysfunction, a posterior-superior axis, and a lateral atlas subluxation.

I told the Mom, "I'm not sure this is the cause of the hematoma, but truly it is never a good idea to leave this kind of stress in the spine – especially while his body is trying to heal and grow. From the looks of the video, there is a very high probability that the mal-positioning of the top two vertebrae were caused by the wrenching of the neck during the birthing process. It also appeared as if there were not really any other options at the time."

Within two weeks of checking and adjusting this child – axis first, as I was taught – the hematoma was completely gone. Once again, I was amazed by the healing ability of the body – how wonderful! I hope I am here to see the day parking lots are filled with mothers waiting in line to have their babies checked by Chiropractors as they are released from the hospital. In the mean time, I will continue wishing and trying to make this happen.

A very special note to the author of *Well Adjusted Babies*, by Dr. Jennifer Barham–Floreani; thanks to her, Chiropractors have an abundance of research and studies to read and gain confidence from, to teach and share with their patients and the parents of today's children.

Imagine having had the following information at your fingertips – what this will do for your confidence as a practitioner, as well as for the future of children?

Gastaldo found, "Even after vaginal births, 4.6 percent of term babies suffer unexplained brain bleeds and up to 10 percent suffer brain inflammation. The pathologies may possibly be avoided by decreasing distortion of foetal skulls from (a mother's) pelvic misalignments at delivery."

Gutmann explains, "The trauma from the birth process remains an under-publicized, and therefore significantly under-treated problem."

Abraham Towbin, A Harvard University pathologist, found evidence of common spinal injury as a result of the birthing process, including: intracranial hemorrhage, brain contusion, damage to the nerves that govern respiration and vertebral subluxation.

Twin thirteen-year-old pre-pubescent boys, both in remedial classes at school were brought to me by their mother. She had been treated in our office after suffering for many years from low back pain. The boys were suffering from delayed developmental social and intellectual growth. Thank God they had each other! The mother relayed to me there was trauma during their birth – both born with high forceps, a technique used during vaginal delivery when a baby's head is not yet engaged. Their overall development had been delayed from the beginning: late to hold up their heads, slow to begin crawling, difficulty learning to walk and talk.

They were wonderful boys and they made me laugh. I loved their spirit and knew in my heart they were both very intelligent. I took x-rays of their necks that revealed a cervical kyphosis, a complete reversal of the normal lordotic curvature in both of the boy's cervical spines. In addition, both had definite subluxation at the atlas-axis junction.

Within six months of adjusting them, they were integrated into the normal academic curriculum and graduated on to high school. No doubt they still had challenges with feeling as if they were different, however, their lives are changed forever from being adjusted. What if the mother had not asked me to take a look – would I have had the courage to tell her about Chiropractic and the ramifications of the damage caused during the birth?

The most recent blessing to appear in my office, a little eight-year-old boy who just did *not* know how to focus or behave. Full of frustration and anger, he simply could not control himself. A day didn't go by that he wasn't in trouble at school. The mother spent every single day of this child's life trying to reason with him, console him, and teach him how to *behave.* Many people suggested for him to take medication, yet Mom knew in her heart medications were not the answer. Masking a problem was not within her system of beliefs. She thought their suggestion for the use of medication was merely their attempt to make dealing with him easier for themselves, rather than to truly help him.

As a relief, the boy's teacher suggested to try a Chiropractor, and specifically recommended me. The mother was afraid, for many reasons. She heard 'horror' stories about Chiropractic, and truly did not know what to expect. She emailed our clinic and then came to talk with me in a consultation before feeling comfortable enough to bring him in for an examination. To both of our delight, we made a great connection and trust began to develop.

Upon his first visit, I couldn't believe what I felt when I put my hands on his neck: tension at the top, stiffness throughout, and asymmetry with the occiput – as if it had been pushed inward. It took quite an effort for this little boy to even allow me touch him. I asked the mother about his birth.

She explained, "His birthing process was long. I was induced, and after twenty-four hours at an eight centimeter dilation, they decided to perform an emergency c-section. When he was born, the right side of his head was caved-in, and remained that way for the past eight years." She paused, and then added, "He complains of having stomach aches almost every day; it's been several years now."

We performed an sEMG and thermography, revealing significant lesions in the upper cervical and thoracic spine. The severity of his condition displayed in the imaging helped to communicate the significance of its affects on the child's life. When I told the family of his prognosis and the recommended approach to his care, the boy listened and a glow of hope illuminated in his eyes with the realization that his life was about to improve.

A week and a half into the treatment he showed-up at my office with a Christmas stocking he made for me. He smiled and handed it to me, and it hung on my door for the three weeks leading up to Christmas.

After being adjusted, he is a very different person. He and I became very close since his first visit; all along he sensed I understood.

As an added bonus improvement for him, his stomach-aches (that most thought were psychosomatic) were gone. I believe his body was compensating at T5-T6, the segmentally related area of the spine that supplies the stomach. His presentation was somatovisceral. Though most of his ailments are improved, he still has his moments of behavioral difficulty, particularly during a growth spurt. We make sure he is checked a little more frequently during those times.

Why Do We Check And Adjust Our Own Children, Yet Not Always Offer The Same Service To Others?

I did not intend to write entirely on Chiropractic and children, but this area of practice has always tugged at my heartstrings. In 1997, with the help of the most amazing midwife, I gave birth at home to my beautiful daughter Mckenna. My midwife's experience spans the delivery of over 2,000 babies.

Unlucky for us, during delivery Mckenna had the umbilical cord wrapped around her neck three times. Until that moment, I had never seen anybody work so fast in my entire life; the midwife unraveled the cord from around Mckenna's neck faster than the speed of love. A very dear colleague and friend adjusted Mckenna less than an hour after her birth.

I know I was given this child so I could take great care of her. I remember one day when she was about six weeks old, she was crying uncontrollably – way more intensely than any baby normally cries. I looked at my Mom and told her I was scared and I felt like I lost my confidence to check and adjust my own baby. What if it didn't work?

My Mom so gently guided me and said, "Dear, close your eyes and pretend this is just another baby in your clinic, one that you have adjusted many times."

I closed my eyes and adjusted Mckenna, and within minutes she started to settle down. Not a day passes without thinking about the truth of her being born to me, a Chiropractor. I often wonder what her life would be like if she was without a skillful midwife to deliver her, or if she was not checked for subluxation soon after birth. I know I am not only here to love and support her in life, but she is here for me to gain wisdom from. Adjusting a child throughout their stages of life helps knowing with *certainty* an adjustment corrects the body's function. Additionally, watching them grow as they are being adjusted provides a passionate understanding and acknowledgement of the effectiveness an adjustment has on maintaining their body's systems. If birth traumas remain untreated, it is difficult to predict the ramifications they may have on a child's life.

Whether my young friend's development of leukemia was due to a stress at birth, or a reaction to a medication or vaccine, I thoughtfully consider how Chiropractic might have influenced his outcome. What if he was adjusted at birth, or during the stages when leukemia took over his life? I don't know Chiropractic would have undoubtedly changed his situation, yet I cannot say it would not have, either. I know of many people whose lives *have* been changed for the better because of just one adjustment. As for those that went without: maybe they could have lived a little longer; maybe they would not have developed cancer; maybe they would have been strong enough to treat their spouse a little nicer; or maybe they felt in harmony within themselves, reflecting a smile to brighten someone else's day? We can only wonder.

Once upon a time, there was a wise man that used to go to the ocean to do his writing. He had a habit of walking on the beach before he began his work. One day he was walking along the shore. As he looked down the beach, he saw a human figure moving like a dancer. He smiled to himself to think of someone who would dance to the day. So he began to walk faster to catch up. As he got closer, he saw that it was a young man and the young man wasn't dancing, but instead he was reaching down to the shore, picking up something and very gently throwing it into the ocean.

As he got closer, he called out, "Good morning! What are you doing?"

The young man paused, looked up and replied, "Throwing starfish into the ocean."

"I guess I should have asked, why are you throwing starfish into the ocean?"

"The sun is up and the tide is going out. And if I don't throw them in they'll die."

"But young man, don't you realize that there are miles and miles of beach and starfish all along it. You can't possibly make a difference!"

The young man listened politely. Then bent-down, picked up another starfish and threw it into the sea, past the breaking waves. "It made a difference for that one!"

All day long as he wrote, the image of the young man haunted him. He tried to ignore it, but the vision persisted. Finally, late in the afternoon he realized that he the scientist, he the poet, had missed out on the essential nature of the young man's actions. Because he realized that what the young man was doing was choosing not to be an observer in the universe and make a difference. He was embarrassed.

That night he went to bed troubled. When the morning came he awoke knowing that he had to do something. So he got up, put on his clothes, went to the beach and found the young man. And with him he spent the rest of the morning throwing starfish into the ocean. You see, what that young man's actions represent is something that is special in each and every one of us. We have all been gifted with the ability to make a difference. And if we can, like that young man, become aware of that gift, we gain through the strength of our vision the power to shape the future.

~ Re-told by Joel Barker, *The Power of Vision,* 1990. Originally written by Loren Eiseley (1907-1977), *Unexpected Universe,* 1969.

This story has lived inside of me for years – realizing that doing just one thing can make an amazing difference, and we will never truly understand the full impact of that one thing. Knowing there is a gift inside each of us, and finding it is part of our purpose on this earth. Honouring that gift is being truthful to one's self.

So, what drives a person with an inner quest? What motivates a person to rise at 5:15 AM to take a newborn to the office after only four hours sleep? What causes a person to miss family dinners and their child's dance recitals? My drive is sparked to answer the real question, "WHY?" For me, my passion to help children and people keeps my drive alive, and has for many years. I seek for the answers to why they might not be at their best in the first place, and create a path for betterment. This drive within helped me to be a better Mom, a better Chiropractor, a better coach, a better daughter, and hopefully a better person in general. I hope that this helps you find your *why*, or in the very least helps you to identify that you have one, and to search tirelessly for it within you.

Chiropractic is the best-kept secret, although keeping it secret is a sin! I am so thankful for the chance to share a little of my life's journey.

One cannot lead a life that is truly excellent without feeling that one belongs to something greater and more permanent than oneself.
~ *Mihaly Csikszentmihalyi*

- **Health exists when the normally constructed body properly performs its functions.**
- **We do not need to fully understand our passion but to act on it.**
- **What drives you?**
- **Being strongly pulled in a direction.**

Let's Talk Innate

Dr. Lise Cloutier

When I first received the email from Dr. Liz about this book project, my first instinct was "Whoa! I'm so busy with the kids right now, there's no way I can commit time to writing a chapter for a book, especially with a five week deadline!"

My eldest was just starting an out-of-town tournament and hockey playoffs, which last three weeks. Any hockey parent will tell you what it's like during playoffs. Between travel to and from games and the time spent at the rink, there's not much time for anything else. Plus Pierce is a goalie, meaning we need extra time to suit him with the extra gear and padding he wears. On top of that, I had an upcoming seminar to prepare for and our nanny/housekeeper was leaving to go home to the Philippines for five weeks to get married. Totally bad timing, right?

The interesting part though, is the day before receiving Dr. Liz's email I told my husband I was feeling a bit "blah" recently. A combination of being so focused on juggling work, home and the children's busy schedules had left me feeling stagnant in the area of personal growth. For me, personal growth is a fundamental need, kind of like food, water and exercise, that I must pursue on an on-going basis to feel fulfilled in my day-to-day life. So, the timing was actually naturally-right. Besides, I was being asked to write on behalf of innate intelligence; how hard could it be? When something is meant to be, innate will always provide the time and resources somehow, someway. I just had to trust Universal Principles for this project, like I trust for the other aspect of my life.

Let's Talk Innate

How do I begin talking about innate? First, I believe innate is expressed on a few different levels: the physical, mental and spiritual. When a person is 100 percent connected to his/her innate powers on all three levels, everything naturally flows. Everything in your life becomes easy and effortless and you're living life in the *sweet spot*. Two examples of flourishing with innate are a professional athlete giving a peak-career and flawless Olympic gold medal performance and an artist creating a most *ah-inspiring* masterpiece. In the Chiropractic practice, it's being totally in the *zone*, effortlessly yet intently focusing on every patient adjustment and getting out of the way for healing miracles to occur left, right and center.

As a Chiropractor, you know you are connected when you have full *PTC* (present-time-consciousness) and you innately know where to place your hands without even thinking about it. The coolest element about the work we do as Chiropractors is removing interferences for innate to flow. We know when the human mind, body and spirit are aligned, the body is able to express optimal innate intelligence; meaning an individual will be on their authentic journey doing exactly what it is they are destined to pursue and/or achieve in life – whether that means being the best parent, doctor, teacher, architect, artist or athlete. Everyday, I am blessed with the privilege of performing the power of a Chiropractic adjustment, to tap into and maximize my patients' innate, inborn potential so they may share their optimal authenticity through innate expression. This allows them to maximize their experiences, their learning, their skill development, their love and compassion wherever their life journey takes them. This is why I love Chiropractic so much! With Chiropractic, I have the opportunity to see people blossom on all levels in front of my very eyes.

Being Chosen Is An Honor And A Gift

As a Chiropractor, I truly have one of the best jobs in the entire whole-wide world. To be *chosen* to be a Chiropractor is seriously such a privilege, an honor and a gift. As a speaker and coach in the realm of Chiropractic, I sometimes become so frustrated with the Chiropractors who struggle in practice. It seems they fail to understand or have lost sight of the fundamental Principles of innate as they pertain to health and healing. My friends and colleagues out there, Chiropractic is EASY! Let's stop making it so complicated. We truly have the best career in the Universe. I really can't think of any other profession that taps into the human potential to the level and extent we do. Trust in innate and the gift of healing in your hands.

Innate Miracles In Practice

In my fifteen years in practice, I've had the opportunity to witness and observe so many miracles and transformations. Some were mere instantaneous, like the week-old newborn brought to me by his grandmother; he had not had a bowel movement in five days and was in respiratory distress. Within seconds of the adjustment, we observed a notable physiological response in the baby's breathing pattern, followed by a huge bowel movement within a minute or two. How do you spell relief in an infant who has not had a bowel movement in five days? By the way, Doris, the grandmother, only brought him to me because she understood the detrimental impact of subluxations from the birthing process. If you want these types of referrals in your practice, it is crucial to take the time to properly educate your patients on the causes and consequences of subluxation on the human frame.

A miracle occurred early on in practice. An eleven-year-old boy from Belarus was referred to me by his father. Allow me to elaborate on this story, as it is an interesting one. The father was a janitor who came into my office looking for help with his back pain. After a few weeks of adjusting him, he sat up from the table one afternoon and looked me squarely in the eyes. In his best broken English, asked me if I could possibly help his son. The most interesting part was the way he posed the question, because it was more like he had an epiphany, as if my services were possibly the answer to his prayers to help his son.

When I asked him what was wrong, he told me his son had not been able to speak since birth and not a single doctor or specialist was able to help him. The only clue he was offered was that due to a difficult and lengthy childbirth, it appeared his son had sustained damage from lack of oxygen to his brain. Additionally, since his family had moved to Canada, doctors put him on *Ritalin*, explaining his speech impediment was due to ADHD. The father did not feel this was the answer.

Without hesitation, I looked at the dad and told him if his son had subluxation in the upper part of his neck, chances were I could help. As I finished escorting him to the front desk to help him schedule a check-up for his son, my first thought was, "Whoa, what did I just say? Chances are I *can't* help this child if he's been brain damaged!"

You see, I'd only been in practice for just over a year. Therefore my certainty, conviction and belief in Chiropractic were not quite at an all time high. As if innate had made me utter those words out of nowhere, I didn't know where they came from.

Low and behold, the boy came in for his check-up, and what did I find? A subluxated atlas! My educated brain kicked-in, thinking, "What a relief! At least I have something to work with."

So, I started adjusting this young boy three times per week. I adjusted his full spine, but initially focused on his atlas. Three weeks passed by, then five, and no change whatsoever. On an afternoon in the sixth week, I entered into the adjusting room and his entire family was in the room, with a *buzz* circulating the air. I thought it was a little unusual, as he had previously only come in with his father.

The sixteen-year-old sister proceeded telling me her younger brother started speaking earlier in the day. *Wow!* Talk about a celebration, and a major boost for my belief, certainty and conviction in Chiropractic. I can't speak for my fellow colleagues, but there were many days, especially early in my practice when the little voice in the back of my mind doubted whether I was truly making a difference in people's health and lives with Chiropractic. In fact, I spent several hours a week praying and meditating for miracles to happen in the lives of my patients to strengthen my beliefs of the Chiropractic Principles. Well, there were miracles for sure.

To offer further evidence of how Chiropractic impacts lives, let me tell you of another event in my practice that blew me away. I started adjusting a thirty-two-year-old female suffering from headaches and neck pain. During her health history, she disclosed that she had a pretty "rough" childhood, and was coming out of a bad relationship, but failed to elaborate on details.

Being young and inexperienced at the time, I decided not to press her for details. Again, my educated mind reminded me I wasn't a psychologist and I should stay focused on the spine and nervous system. (In hindsight, for this particular case, staying focused on the nervous system was the best thing I could have done).

Long story short, about a month into her care, she sat up after being adjusted and unexpectedly gave me the biggest hug ever, and said, "Thank you for saving my life."

Shocked, I said, "What do you mean?"

She began telling me prior to the start of her care she was in a serious state of depression and had contemplated suicide. When she started receiving adjustments, she reconnected to her innate source and the veil of darkness slowly lifted; she regained control and hope in her life.

Borrow The Experience Of Others To Gain It Yourself

Perhaps you are reading this right now and you are still a student in Chiropractic school, or you have just recently graduated and have not yet had the chance to witness or experience the power of an adjustment. You may even be thinking, "Okay, this lady is crazy!"

If I may share a piece or two of advice for a successful career in Chiropractic:

1) Take time out of your schedule to observe successful Chiropractors during prime time in their practices.
2) Read as many Chiropractic success stories, miracles, testimonials, as you can possibly manage. Many Chiropractors collect them and through your experience, so can you.
3) Chiropractic seminars/conferences are a must! If you are going to attend only one or two a year, be sure to attend one with plenty of Chiropractic Philosophy and Principles.

We can never review enough philosophy. With exposure to it, a new aspect will click in your brain and cause growth in your practice. Every time I attend a seminar including philosophy, at least, I've seen growth within my practice. The tips I shared are an opportunity for gaining the certainty and conviction needed to succeed in practice.

I forgot to mention, the best Chiropractors are those able to communicate the message with ease. Therefore, if communication and public speaking are not your forte, I urge you to join a speaking group such as toastmasters – available in just about every community around the globe.

Become Comfortable Speaking As You Educate Others

Speaking about certainty, conviction and communication reminds me of a conversation I recently had with my exam doctor. We have a policy in our office: at the end of every week, each staff member must hand in a communication sheet about the good and bad of the week, goals achieved or challenges faced. A few weeks ago, my exam Doctor left me a note saying he was having a hard time learning his scripts.

My response to him, "Keep repeating the scripts over and over until you *own* them." When you can speak with certainty and conviction, there will be no objections from patients. They will clearly understand the devastating impact of subluxations on their health and how that plays out in their lives. Most importantly the patients will understand your intent. We just have to think of actors for a minute. How often do actors rehearse scripts, tones, and gestures to embody extreme overjoy, insane sadness or terrifying fear? They create a human emotional connection with viewers for the sole purpose of entertainment. We, as Chiropractors, do it to reshape lives.

Vitalism And My Family

If you are a vitalistic individual, there's nothing like parenthood to test your beliefs. For me, it started when I became pregnant with our first child back in 1998. I had the entire pregnancy and birthing process planned out. I hired a midwife, a doula and everything was going to go "perfectly" for us to have a home birth. The goal was to give birth in the most natural way possible, the way it was always intended to be. I definitely wanted to stay as far away from the medical setting as possible, because *their way* of handling the birthing process is the furthest thing from love and innate wisdom. In fact, being the vitalistic person I am, I believe their procedures and techniques are questionably barbaric.

Unfortunately, innate had other plans. In my thirty-third week of pregnancy, on a very busy day at the office, our unborn son, Pierce, decided to turn head up. For the next seven weeks we tried everything under the sun to encourage him to turn back around into the position necessary for a vaginal birth. To our disappointment, nothing worked, not even the breech Webster technique that has worked and still works very well on many of our Chiropractic patients. Time had run out, and the reality was that he was big (almost ten pounds) and I was sporting a basketball belly. Long story short, my midwife informed me we would have to do a hospital birth and to come prepared with a birthing plan if we were still wanting to do this as natural as possible. I immediately wrote out my birthing plan and prepared myself for battle.

Shortly after we arrived to the hospital, I was assessed by an obgyn. I won't mention any names, but let me tell you about her bedside manner. My initial introduction to her was when she strolled into my hospital room unannounced, wheeling in a cart containing equipment to monitor the baby. She never introduced herself; she was on a mission to do her procedure and did not seem to care about anything else. She definitely did not show my husband or me any care, concern, or support – especially for a first-time laboring mother. However, she was aware my unborn child was in a breech position, and when I enthusiastically shared with her my "as natural as possible" birthing plan, she looked at me as if I had three heads, and asked me if I was trying to purposely kill my unborn child. Needless to say, my husband and I were less than impressed with her lack of support and professionalism.

After that brief conversation, it became very clear to me the lack of understanding from the medical profession of Universal Principles as they pertain to health. It is sad they

have become so dependent on prescription drugs and surgeries they fail to remember the fundamental Principles of
health and healing. They have forgotten to trust in the innate
wisdom of the human body and what it is capable of doing.
There is a happy ending to my story, however. By the time I
was ready to deliver Pierce, the "I don't believe in nature or
innate" obgyn was no longer on duty. She was replaced by a
lovely Greek doctor open to allowing me to try to naturally
deliver Pierce. Sure enough, after fifty-four minutes of pushing, Pierce was born, butt first but otherwise perfectly
healthy. Today, Pierce is ten-years-old, weighs one hundred
pounds, and five feet and one inch tall. He is fully bilingual
and does very well in school. He is a fantastic goaltender in
hockey and also plays basketball and snowboards. This
summer he is looking forward to playing football and he
eventually wants to become an actor and/or pyrotechnician.

Our second blessing came on November 1, 2003 when
our second son, Noah, was born at home. His childbirth was
very easy, I might add. He is a six-year-old budding ball of
energy and as sharp as a tack. He loves *Lego's*, videogames, is
fascinated with anything military and loves to pull pranks.
His wicked sense of humor is infectious. Our children are so
different from one another, and every day they teach me new
and wonderful things about their understanding of innate.
They have both received regular Chiropractic care since they
were born, making them so in tune with themselves and the
world they live in. Whatever their journey, I know they will
grow up to be the best they can be.

Children Are Already Tuned-In, Stay That Way

Children are so much more connected to their innate than
adults. It seems the older we become, the more the educated
mind gets in the way and the more stressors we have in our
lives. It becomes more difficult to stay tuned and connected

to our innate, and is something we all need to work at every day. In the stressful world we live in currently, I really see this as the challenge Chiropractors are faced with. On an on-going basis we need to address lifestyle stressors whether physical, chemical, or mental/emotional. Helping our patients develop strategies and solutions to overcome these stressors is a key for them to reconnect to their innate source and help them express their optimal potential.

- **Respect the honor and gift of being chosen to do what you do.**
- **Look for and witness miracles.**
- **Borrow the experience of others to gain it yourself.**
- **Become comfortable speaking as you educate others.**
- **Sometimes the Universe has other plans.**

How Chiropractic Changed My Life
Dr. Marlene Turner

A journey of a thousand miles begins with a single step.
~ Chinese Proverb

My mother was slated for surgery, both wrists: Carpal Tunnel Syndrome.

We all have experienced those times in life when someone we love is in pain. My mother had severe neck pain and pins and needles in her hands for years. I remember seeing her reading at the kitchen table at 2:30 AM because the pain kept her awake. She was losing sleep, losing energy and losing her zest for life. She was forty-five-years-old. As her daughter, this was a hard thing to watch and I wished I could do something to help her. I felt so helpless. Her friend heard about a Chiropractor that said he might be able to help. So, *as a last resort,* my mother had scheduled her first appointment. She was scared, skeptical and at the same time, she felt she had nothing to lose. So she tried it out.

As her Chiropractic adjustments progressed throughout the weeks and months to follow, we saw a dramatic change in her condition. She was rested, happy, and smiling. She had her energy back. She felt like a new woman.

This begins my story of how Chiropractic changed my mother's life, my life, and the lives of many others.

I did not want to go to the Chiropractor. "I was fine." I had just a little bit of low back pain from bending and lifting at my summer job in the grocery store, nothing serious. My mother wanted me to see her Chiropractor because she was so thrilled with her care. She was so adamant about it I basically just went to please her. Little did I know, giving into her wishes created a life defining moment for me. I was eighteen-years-old.

Many people think Chiropractic is just about resolving back pain and neck pain, just for pain to go away. That's what I thought too, until something happened to me on my tenth Chiropractic visit. I might sound crazy, but a veil of fog was lifted from my brain – I could think more clearly, concentrate better and I had so much more energy. I felt much more *alive*. I used to see my Chiropractor early in the morning, and then head off to university to swim lengths in the pool. I felt like I could swim effortlessly, forever – a feeling I will never forget. The funny part, I didn't know I had this veil of fog until it was gone. I didn't know I had low energy until I had much more.

What if I never went to that Chiropractor thirty-seven years ago? What would my life look like now? I shudder to think...

My experience was so powerful I told my friends in university about it and suggested they switch fields of study to become Chiropractors. I just loved my new energized life, and I never had a doctor who cared so much and was so interested in me. I tried to set up interviews with my friends and my Chiropractor to discuss a Chiropractic career, but they just were not excited.

A Ship Without A Rudder

I kind of floated along in life, not really sure of my destiny. I scraped by in high school with only the minimum grades necessary to enter university. Come to think of it, I only went to university because all my friends were going and I didn't know what else to do. At that time it seemed like a life sentence of uncertainty for me. I fell into psychology, then criminology. I knew the credits I accumulated as an art student could not be transferred over to science, so I continued along in my criminology studies. A Chiropractic career for me was not in the cards, or so I thought.

I applied to graduate school to become a criminologist. I was not accepted and I was devastated! I then fell into becoming a teacher, because I really didn't know what else to do. To be honest, the primary reason I changed universities was because my boyfriend at the time was attending Queen's University where the teaching program was offered. How's that for a lame reason?

While earning my teaching degree I worked in a prison for women to gather more criminology experience. I received my teaching degree and began teaching for the Ministry of Corrections in a juvenile detention center. I loved the offenders, but I did not love the job. I knew something was missing.

Then, in a moment when I least expected it, my life changed.

Destiny

During a visit to my Chiropractor, I said to him, "If I had to do it all over again, I would be a Chiropractor."

His response was, " Why don't you?"

I relayed my thoughts, "I've already spent four years of university in arts, not science, and I am too old."

"How old are you?"

"Twenty-three."

His response was, " I was twenty-four when I started."

A light bulb went on in my head. Something shifted. *In that moment,* I knew I would become a Chiropractor. I *knew.* It's hard to explain that feeling. It came with the greatest sense of urgency, a sense I couldn't wait to start. I had to do it right then. When I made that instantaneous decision, the Universe shifted in response. Life just seemed to fall into place. There were many obstacles to overcome, such as going back to school for an additional five years in order to transition from teacher to being a Chiropractor. But it all seemed to flow effortlessly.

I have met many patients over the years that are working at jobs they do not like. Many patients who are students have approached me because they have no idea what they want to do with their lives. I tell them my story in hope to motivate them in some way, to help them along the path they are destined to follow.

I tell you that story to share my insights:

1. Things happen for a reason. I was not accepted into graduate school for a reason. I did not continue with teaching for a reason. And there was a reason I saw my Chiropractor that day.

2. Never give up, even when things don't seem to be going your way, move forward, stay the course, and be open to new ideas and to change.

3. Never underestimate the words you say. "We never know how far reaching something we may think, say or do today, will effect the lives of millions tomorrow." ~ B.J. Palmer DC, Developer of Chiropractic.

4. "I started at age twenty-four." Those words changed my life and the lives of thousands.

5. Listen to the small voice within. I did not listen to my inner voice. Deep down I knew I would love to be a Chiropractor, but I never acknowledged it. If something excites you, pay attention.

6. Your life can change in the blink of an eye.

The Greatest Gift

I don't know what your destiny will be, but one thing I know, as philosopher Albert Schweitzer said, "The only ones among you who will be really happy are those who will have sought and found how to serve."

End of story? Actually, no.

I was so excited to begin practice, the months and years went by and believe it or not, I found my career very unfulfilling. For *six years* I felt isolated and alone in my profession. I did not feel I was making a difference in peoples' lives. "Is this it? Is this what I spent all those years in school for?" I asked myself many times over. I was unhappy with my career. Little did I know, out of my greatest despair was to come my greatest gift.

I had been operating what I call a *pain relief* type of practice. Patients came in with a painful condition, were adjusted, and didn't come back until they had pain again. That certainly wasn't the kind of Chiropractic care I had received, but I was afraid to tell my patients the truth of Chiropractic. Yes, afraid. Chiropractic was not being accepted by mainstream medicine at the time, and wasn't particularly popular (not that it is now). I found myself going along with the medical model of disease and just cared for patients from a symptomatic point of view. And, I was unhappy doing it.

That all changed the day I met one of my mentors, Dr. James Carter. Dr. Carter is a Chiropractor, and for years he inspired Chiropractors all over the world. He rekindled the fire and passion within me and taught me far more about Chiropractic than I ever knew before. I became obsessed with my new mission of helping as many people as I could through Chiropractic. He and my colleagues supported me through the transition of finally speaking the whole truth about Chiropractic. I learned patients deserve to know and need to know when we work with the whole person and remove nerve interference from the spinal nerves we see incredible changes in peoples' lives – mentally, physically, and spiritually. If there is interference to the master control system of the body, the brain and spinal nerves, then the body cannot function at 100 percent of its capacity. It will function at less than optimum: less health, less life, more *dis*-ease. Everyone deserves to experience the best health possible. Chiropractic and the Chiropractic healthy lifestyle can help achieve it.

Until the day I met Dr. Carter, I was not speaking the truth. I was in fear of speaking what was in my heart. I was playing life small. Nelson Mandela's speech could have been written for me:

> Our deepest fear is not that we are inadequate. Our deepest fear is that we are powerful beyond measure. It is our light, not our darkness, that most frightens us. We ask ourselves, who am I to be brilliant, gorgeous, talented, and fabulous? Actually, who are you not to be? You are a child of God. Your playing small doesn't serve the world. There's nothing enlightened about shrinking so that other people won't feel insecure around you. We are all meant to shine, as children do. We are born to make manifest the glory of God that is within us. It's not just in some of us; it's in everyone. And as we let our own light shine, we unconsciously give other people permission to do the same. As we are liberated from our own fear, our presence automatically liberates others.
> ~ *Nelson Mandela, Inaugural Speech, 1994*

When listening to my inner voice about becoming a Chiropractor, my destiny changed. We become unstoppable when our purpose becomes clear. I was not *playing small* anymore. As I was liberated from my own fear of speaking the truth, others' lives would be liberated also. As I was liberated from my fear, miracles began to occur in my personal life and in my professional life.

Liberated

Change always comes bearing gifts.
~ *Price Pritchett*

In my personal life, the first miracle presented itself. I gave birth to twins. Boys. The second (or perhaps third) miracle occurred twenty months later – my daughter was born. Three children under the age of two: now, that's a lot of diapers! For someone told by doctors there was a 16 percent chance of conceiving – that's a lot of babies at once. (Just for the record, six years later I had a fourth baby.) Busy with three babies and a very successful practice, this wasn't playing small. While caring for my children, explosive changes were occurring in my professional life.

My practice had literally changed overnight. Once I decided to share my truth, I walked into my office the next day a different person. The Universe responded. Our Chiropractic practice skyrocketed from 200 patient visits per week to 550 patient visits per week, in only ten weeks. Chiropractors who have their own office will appreciate the significance of this challenge. Can you imagine what it would be like for you if your already successful business more than doubled in ten weeks? Our staff and office procedures remained the same. To be clear, I did nothing differently, but *I* was different. And that made all the difference. The change occurred because I shifted my thinking. I made the decision to *tell the Chiropractic story.*

Because we more than doubled our practice in a short period of time, our office was in absolute chaos. I was so desperate, I quickly recruited my next-door neighbor to come in and help with the additional paperwork. My CHA (Chiropractic health assistant) wanted to put lawn chairs out on the sidewalk for people to sit on because the reception area was so busy. It was insane. We were excited and our patients were excited.

Over time, we gained order to our procedures and systems and the office was more organized with great patient flow. Never a doubt, those patients were served the best Chiropractic care. After all, who doesn't want to be adjusted by an inspired, passionate doctor surrounded by motivated staff in a loving office?

I tell you that story to point out inner happiness is the fuel of success. Once we decide to honour ourselves and tell *our* truth, then all else follows. Making the decision is the first step. When we decide, the Universe moves to allow our truth to become reality.

As B.J. Palmer said, "Get the big idea, all else follows." The big idea for me was to tell the truth about Chiropractic. Don't hold back, don't be afraid, just accept that it will be okay. For me, all else *did* follow. The biggest mind shift in my life appeared, and it affected every decision I made: how I raised my children, my way of life, and what I, as a person, stand for to this day.

The Balancing Act

Happiness is when what you think, what you say, and what you do are in harmony.
~ *Mahatma Gandhi*

In speaking with many professionals over the years, a good percentage of them women, many have difficulty balancing parental and career responsibilities. I remember one patient in particular who had been a lawyer for five years before her first child was born. When her baby was one-year-old, she said to me, "You know, Dr. Turner, I don't feel I'm filling either role very well. I'm not practicing law well and I'm not being the best mom I can be."

It seemed so sad to me – we need to find the balance, we need to find what works for us. We *can* have our cake and eat it, too. Dr. James Carter helped me reveal how to make it work for me.

The first thing he suggested was for Chiropractors to understand the Law of Present Time Consciousness. What does that mean? It means, when you are with your patients, be *with* your patients: focus 100 percent on them, on the adjustment, and on your intention. Don't be thinking about your next fishing trip or what to cook for dinner. Rather, be totally present in the here and now. As you are reading this book, are you present 100 percent? Or are you thinking about your next vacation? When we are totally present we laser in, we experience more in less time.

Time x Intensity = Results

Dr. John Demartini, an incredible Chiropractor, spiritual teacher and author, taught me that if we increase the intensity (i.e. increase our focus), then we decrease the time it takes to get the results we desire. Being totally present with our patients allows one to get more results in less time - more results than you thought possible. Unfocused, unintentional acts don't usually reap great rewards, but rather, mediocrity.

The same is true in our relationships. If we increase our focus, if we increase our attention on the people we love when we are with them, the quality of our relationships will improve. For example, if we spend an hour with our children and during that time we talk with them while at the same time reading the newspaper, we really aren't doing either activity very well. Wouldn't it be better to spend half an hour with our children, totally focused on them, and then half an hour reading the newspaper? You *and* your children would be more fulfilled.

The Law of Present Time Consciousness directs us to be *with* our children, *with* our patients. This way, we have the time to create the balance we so desperately desire in our lives.

Dr. Carter's second suggestion was to set up a support system to create the opportunity to have the best of both worlds. My husband, a teacher, was enrolled in my vision of telling the Chiropractic story and helping as many people as possible. He is an amazing dad and was willing to do whatever it took for me to be successful.

We hired a nanny/babysitter to come into our home so we could minimize domestic chores when not working. The main objective was when we were not working to be truly spending time with our children.

In the office, it was important for us that our office staff members were on board with our philosophy of Chiropractic, as well as our intention of helping as many people as we could. The role of our Chiropractic health assistants is vital in delivering the message about Chiropractic. Never underestimate the value of a really good Chiropractic assistant. They can make the difference between a mediocre patient experience in the office and an enlightened, uplifting and positive patient experience. They are an invaluable element of the whole- patient healing process.

Our office manager became my personal assistant as well. She too was enrolled in the vision of helping as many people as possible through Chiropractic. We built a strong, cohesive team in the office and we loved it. Our office procedures were streamlined, efficient and allowed for expansion, while at the same time maintaining Chiropractic standards of excellence.

We had financial systems in place so our banking was automatic, and our vacation and tax accounts were streamlined. When tax time and vacation time rolled around, the money was already saved.

Present time consciousness and a great support system are the secrets to balancing a successful career in Chiropractic with family life. Yes, we can find balance. You just have to trust.

> Take the first step in faith. You don't have to see the whole staircase. Just take the first step.
> ~ *Dr. Martin Luther King, Jr.*

Health For All

> He who has health has hope. And he who has hope has everything.
> ~ *Arabian Proverb*

How does what we say and do affect others?

Take Dave for example. He was a fifty-one-year-old male who came into our office complaining of low back pain that he had on and off for twenty years. He was fed up and came in for care. After three weeks his back pain subsided, and on one day he asked the question, "Hey doc, do these adjustments have anything to do with constipation? I have been constipated my entire life, and now I don't have any problems at all. In fact, when I was a young kid my grandfather used to give me a product called *Dynomite*, which seemed to work wonders back then. Since then, I have had to take laxatives my whole life. What does Chiropractic have to do with constipation?"

"Well, if we remove the nerve interference to the bowel, the bowel can function properly." What is the likelihood that Dave would run into other bowel problems as he aged? Maybe polyps, maybe irritable bowel syndrome, maybe colon cancer, who really knows? All I know, Dave is much better off without nerve interference than he is with it.

And what about little Robbie? His mother brought him to me as a last resort. She really didn't know anything about Chiropractic, but she was desperate. He was five months old and as cute as a button. Unfortunately he had been exhibiting severe colic for the entire five months of his young life. He cried uncontrollably for a minimum of twelve hours per day. He only slept in spurts, and his mother was at her wits end. During the consultation (with the baby wailing) I discovered the pregnancy and childbirth was relatively "normal," *except* for the use of forceps during the last stage of delivery. After examining Robbie, I determined he had two areas of nerve interference in his neck, probably caused by the "normal" delivery. Yes, normal deliveries, with or without forceps, can create vertebral misalignments. In fact, the birthing process is one of the most common causes of health issues from birth, throughout life. I adjusted his spine very gently and carefully. I explained to his mother I felt he would need several more adjustments to correct his underlying problem. I never saw that baby again.

Six months later, an individual I had never met before approached me at a back yard barbeque. "I want to thank you for saving our marriage."

I couldn't recall saving anyone's marriage.

The perplexed look on my face prompted him to respond, "I am Robbie's father." Five months of a screaming baby had put such a strain on their relationship they were considering ending their marriage. One adjustment changed the course of their lives.

All I know, Robbie is a lot better off without nerve interference than he is with it – a lot better off at five months old, at five-years-old, and when he becomes fifty-years-old.

Chiropractic is truly amazing. Know, as Chiropractors we sometimes will not be made aware of the far-reaching effect Chiropractic has on our patients. We may not find out about the long- term impact we have on their health and their lives. From the words we say, our caring touch, to the powerful adjustment: it all makes a difference.

And know that you, as patients, and Chiropractic assistants, have the opportunity to help so many people by spreading the truth of Chiropractic around the world. Too few people understand the potential within them, and it is up to us, all of us, to share the Chiropractic message.

Aside from my four children, Chiropractic is the best thing that has happened to me. The day I decided to become a Chiropractor changed my destiny, and what a blessing it has been. I have the privilege of being part of the Chiropractic community, and indeed it is a privilege. I am honoured to be a Chiropractor and I am honoured to have the opportunity to touch peoples' lives.

After almost thirty years of Chiropractic practice, I feel the most important thing for you – the reader – to know: regardless of your occupation: love what you do, surround yourself with what you love, know you have inspired others to live better lives, live your truth, speak your truth, and the Universe will support you.

- **From floundering to full steam ahead.**
- **Face destiny.**
- **Liberate yourself through thoughts and actions.**
- **Always a balancing act.**
- **We become what we focus on.**
- **Know that what you do has a profound impact.**

Anything, Nothing, Everything
Dr. Madeline Behrendt

Anything

Cara burst into my office as if arriving at a shoe sale. She is holding, clutching, a card-sized blue envelope.

In the moment a person presents, anticipation meets adrenaline.

The traveler is looking for a change; I'm looking. My senses attune, information exchanges, connections ignite and trusts first steps amble.

Put together carefully, perfectly, in designer logos and fancy lips, Cara's public image assumes success.

She doesn't fool me at all. Pretty clothes can't hide spinal dysfunction, and I shred camouflage to lock on clues that mean trouble: chin rotated left... attached to a head tilted right... connected to uneven shoulders.

After welcoming her, we start making our way through the stack of intake documentation, and develop a rhythm: I ask questions and Cara fidgets with her envelope. Then slowly, she stands up and extends the blue mystery towards me, whispering: "I can't do this."

I look inside and understand her.

What makes a woman's world smaller, darker, and un-controllable?

A body that breaks down, and in my role I witness the betrayed.

Cara will not go to parks anymore, she zigzags the morning route to work and shops for food only late at night. She re-wired the world to avoid babies. Except she cannot avoid her in-laws "Summer Family Extravaganza" invite.

The world is not always gentle to women with reproductive struggles; infertility's strain has boldly altered history, alliances, and life spans - King Henry VIII beheaded Ann Boleyn.

Cara's in-laws do not tolerate failure, especially biological, and they are skilled in emotional and social execution. For two years, Cara had multiple assisted interventions, trying so hard to deliver a baby, with no success. Neither money nor will were a barrier, so she tried *anything* – a very long list. I was a pit stop on what she called her "tour of desperation."

At this point, some might offer Cara their own brand of hope. But to me, hope is something best reserved for skinny jeans, parking spaces, and morning hair. "Hope" is not enough for a woman that needs to get well.

So I offer Cara health.

"Insulted," I explained. "Your health becomes insulted from stresses: physical-chemical-mental-emotional." Cara nodded her head yes, yes. "When your body can no longer adapt, the overload can cause interference in the nervous system – and you don't want that."

Mention nervous system and people are all about *location*; what they miss is the real story, *occupation* – as the nervous system directs and controls all functions of the body. Interference is the villain, because function interrupted can result in *dys*-function. And you will not like that.

Think of interference as the biggest, *baddest* football player chasing you down; and then, apply truly vicious hits. For *NFL* Hall of Fame wide receiver Jerry Rice, this interference was real. He credits Chiropractic for keeping him in the game and shares his remarkable story as spokesman for the Foundation for Chiropractic Progress.

Nerve interference is not good for football and it is not good for fertility.

The good news for Jerry and for Cara is that Chiropractors can detect and correct nerve interference, officially called vertebral subluxation. Great news if you want health.

So I offer Cara Chiropractic.

After all, *why* Cara found me is because I documented the positive response to Chiropractic care among infertile women, regardless of factors including age, history, or previous intervention. *How* she found me is because these findings are part of the fertility world and featured by these trusted resources:

1) **Clinical resources** = San Diego's leading provider of fertility services, the San Diego Fertility Center, included this recommendation in their newsletter:

    > A new combination patients might want to consider is an appointment with the Chiropractor. Recent studies published in the *Journal of Vertebral Subluxation Research (JVSR)* suggested a link between a woman's infertility and nerve interference caused by spinal distortions...Even though the results are not conclusive, it increases awareness of the central nervous system's role in the fertility world.
    > ~ *Miracle News*, March 2004

2) **Advocacy resources** = The National Infertility Association, *Resolve*, extended the honor of inviting me to

contribute the article on Chiropractic care when they devoted an entire issue of their *Family Building Magazine* to the topic Complementary Medicine and Holistic Care.

3) **Media resources** = *CBS-TV* broke the story, followed by *ABC*, and it was a hit with affiliate stations coast to coast: New York, Seattle, Philadelphia, Salt Lake City, Cincinnati, San Antonio, Tucson, Miami, Boise, Raleigh-Durham and more.

4) **Medical resources** = the study also appeared on the sites: the Association for Reproductive Medicine (www.asrm.org), OBGYN.net, and preconception.com.

The catalyst for the excitement about Chiropractic is the retrospective research study I directed exploring the link between Chiropractic care and fertility, "Insult, Interference, and Infertility: An Overview of Chiropractic Research" published May 2, 2003 in the *Journal of Vertebral Subluxation Research (JVSR),* an online peer-reviewed scientific journal.

I designed the study to reflect the variables of practice:
- Eleven Chiropractors contributed: from the U.S., Canada, and Israel
- Ages: ranged from 22 to 65
- Chiropractic techniques utilized: 8
- Time of care: 1 to 20 months
- Presenting concerns: back pain, neck pain
- Stress histories included:
  - Physical (falls, fractured sacrum, motor vehicle accidents)
  - Chemical (colitis, blocked fallopian tubes, diabetes, amenorrhea)
  - Mental/emotional (stress from previous miscarriage, infertility)

Of the fourteen women studied, all were infertile, nine had previous unsuccessful assisted treatments, and four were undergoing assisted treatment concurrent with entering Chiropractic care.

Vertebral subluxations were detected in all the women. Chiropractic care was applied; objective and subjective findings tracked changes in health, as subluxations reduced and function improved. Each of the women became pregnant and delivered a healthy baby.

While more research is needed to further study the link between the central nervous system and fertility, these results may suggest the relationship between structure, nerve function, and fertility is an unrecognized health problem for people with fertility struggles.

Americans are losing the ability to reproduce, a natural function, it is alarming. The National Survey of Family Growth's data reports, "In 2002, an estimated 7.3 million American women ages 15-44 years had impaired fecundity" (i.e. experienced difficulties conceiving or bringing a pregnancy to term during their lifetime).

For all the women struggling with fertility I'm trained to look beyond symptoms to evaluate function. So I offer health. I offer Chiropractic.

Because when I look at statistics, I see people, I see Cara.

Life University inspired me to ask a big question, on my mind as I rushed between dissection, clinic, class, and board prep: "What can I do?"

Parker Seminars *wowed* me, and I kept asking: "What can I do?"

I graduated, opened a practice, got rolling, and found my answer: "Connect women to Chiropractic and Chiropractors to women."

First step: Create "The Role and Relationship of Chiropractic and Women's Health Issues – A Call For Research," published in *JVSR*, 2000. The response confirmed my instincts were correct.

Second step: United Nations. "Perspectives on Chiropractic Care in Women's Health and Quality of Life" presented by the Chiropractic panel of Drs. Veronica Gutierrez, Theresa Warner, myself and the Secretary of the NGO Health Committee, Christopher Kent. Held in conjunction with the NGO sessions during the *45th Annual Assembly of the Commission on the Status of Women*, this event was a first for Chiropractic and truly inspiring.

Third step: *Web*MD. My commentary provided the editor of *Web*MD a Chiropractic resource and I was interviewed for their article "Women Behaving Badly," and one of only a few Chiropractors to appear on this leading medical site.

The next steps take me to Congress, NIH, popular magazines, and more, as women's health issues travel through culture, fashion, research, and policy.

And always back to my practice.

Are you wondering if Cara is pushing a Silver Cross, smooching her tiny, new, pink boss, and healing over past loss? Here's a hint: her in-laws get adjusted, every Tuesday, every Thursday.

More than ever I'm determined to connect women to Chiropractic, Chiropractors to women. Because of anything... because of...

Nothing

The ball crashed off the glass, shot contested, rebound denied, game over.

Victory. The crowd roared. Mom beamed. The coach almost smiled.

Alyssa is a leaping, shot-stopping, force of nature born to win basketball games like a pro. She thrives in a bubble of "Vinsanity," her sneakers, energy drink, and gear endorsed by *NBA* star Vince Carter. At eighteen, this high school star is on a fast track to a future accessible only for *rare* athletes. Expectations? Huge.

Then Alyssa's knees quit playing.

The bubble burst, and her life got very quiet. And slow. Alyssa sucked down aspirin and started treatment - injections in both knees. The first time she hobbled into my reception room, a ninety-year-old patient zoomed right by her.

My specialty started as Women's Wellness, the unexpected result is my practice is full of sports injuries, because women trust me and bring in their kids: athletes who get messed up running, shooting, and scoring. That's *how* Alyssa's mom found me.

Whiplash is *why* she found me. In a high school football player whose neck was the accidental target of the momentum of a much heavier lineman launched offside. His fierce mom took him right off the field to my office. We got to work and the great results made their way around the *Mom* network.

So when her family arrived at my office for their first Chiropractic experience they wondered what I could do. I reassured them my care did not duplicate either treatment and introduced Chiropractic's approach to answering their concerns: drug-free and hands-on.

I explained it is important to evaluate how Alyssa's entire body moves, as knees act because of those connections. My focus is the relationship between spine and function, and I asked directly, "Why'd your knees only last ten years?" Their eyes got big, and the family became very interested in what I would do.

What interference caused Alyssa to go from home-court to home-bound? That is what I relied on the Chiropractic exam to uncover. "Try not to move or speak," I instructed, placing the sensitive sEMG scanners of the Insight Subluxation Station™ directly on the exposed muscles supporting Alyssa's young spine.

"The test is silent, painless, and the alcohol prep feels soothing." Red, green, and blue lines flicked across the screen as the scan recorded the amount of tension in paraspinal muscle activity compared to a normal muscle tonicity. Elevations and deviations identified, the procedure took less than ten minutes.

I utilize surface EMG technology for quantifying the muscular changes associated with vertebral subluxation, first to determine baseline status and then to track changes during care.

The exam continued with posture, asymmetry, and range of motion evaluations. Individual and family medical histories were discussed, stress scores for activities of daily living compiled, and goals identified. All these factors contribute to identifying vertebral subluxations and creating a treatment plan. In addition, I watched Alyssa's highlight reel on *YouTube* to identify any irregularities in movement, and researched the *WNBA* and *NCAA*'s latest findings on basketball injury patterns.

Many people think of pain as a problem located in the epicenter of their hurt. The reality is that the original subluxation can occur anywhere along the spine and result in symptoms elsewhere. Even more disturbing is that degeneration – spine, discs, joints – either slow or aggressive, can be silent until the body's ability to adapt is exhausted. Then in come the noise and the pain.

Alyssa's total results were stunning: this wasn't an injury; it was a reveal.

Her knees were hurting, yes, but the injury really wasn't about her knees. Alyssa's patterns of spinal dysfunction built up enough damage to alter the way her body moved. Poor tracking can affect joints all along the kinetic chain; her knees were just the first unwilling casualties, unable to bear the punishment of repetitive insults.

While this young star could barely process that she wasn't playing this week, I knew much more was at risk. Competitive sports are defined by moments: how an athlete performs at a specific time. Scouts and scholarships are poised at the junction between high school and college.

But a jumper without knees, what kind of offer can she get? *Nothing.* Moment gone, someone grabs your spot and a life turns. At eighteen: *hero* to *has-been.*

For all the *Alyssa's* out there, I feel this. I must ask the questions and provide the care for athletes to repair, to perform. I know the slide from invincible to done is brutal.

Adjusted, Alyssa's now feeling like a champion. End of story? Not exactly.

Sports Chiropractor, celebrity Chiropractor, pediatric Chiropractor, personal injury Chiropractor, wellness Chiropractor – for every life and lifestyle there is a Chiropractor with the skills to deliver care.

For the performer whose nervous system must recover from the stress of traveling and adrenaline overload or a tour could be wrecked; for babies – the tiniest spines with the biggest jobs; or for football players checking out the Professional Football Chiropractic Society to find which Chiropractors the pros go to; Chiropractic care offers a detour off the highway heading from aspirin to operating room-A.

Alyssa's family learned that while an injury is physical, what drives recovery is adding this philosophy: spinal structure drives function. And performance.

Alyssa continues Chiropractic care to promote full expression of her potential; she's added Chiropractic to her playbook.

Adjusted, and that story can mean...

Everything

What if I told you there is a Chiropractic story more popular than news about real electronic brains, or medical stories from the Mayo Clinic and Harvard, is that something you might be interested in? Perhaps that's a story you'd like to create.

Could you? *Would* you?

I did.

I see the Chiropractor as protagonist: trained to serve, battle-tested by health care's flaws, and patrolling her beat in pursuit of promoting life force.

Is this how the world sees Chiropractors? Not sure. I thought it was time.

Of course, every story starts from your own.

I am the daughter of an Irish newspaperman and grew up running around the *New York Times*. I am the granddaughter of a tough Newark Police detective, Sunday suppers with my German grandpa served potato salad and crime lore. Born a Jersey girl, I'd run to the tippy top of my cul-de-sac to stare at New York City's Twin Towers, icons of all that was suppose to be impossible made real, gleaming in the sun. I am a Yankees fan, and madly devoted to the NY Giants since a zygote. NYC is where my soul found its home, inhaling the city's creativity and marking memories all over town. I have survived a lot. Life is good.

And then September 11, 2001 arrived. America attacked.

That day started like any other, by mid-morning, that day started a movement.

Mothers, musicians, clergy, chefs, and Chiropractors asking: "What can we do?"

I asked, as many of you did.

But what?

So I added up my heritage and my history and decided to record history.

Newsman + detective + NY + champion + survivor + Chiropractors = documenting the Chiropractic relief efforts at Ground Zero.

To never forget the lost, honor the relief workers and record the service of Chiropractors. What did they do? What did they say? What really happened?

Because in a time that demanded *everything*, Chiropractic was there.

Do students, training to deliver Chiropractic, know these stories?

Do Chiropractors practicing think about service?

This is what they are missing:

> Groups of police officers stripped their flack jackets off and each dropped a pile of guns at the foot of a Chiropractic bench; it was unsettling to see an arsenal of firearms at the foot of an adjusting table. There were some state troopers who wanted to get adjusted but also wanted to keep their Kevlar vests on. They were guessing that my hands could penetrate where bullets couldn't reach.
>
> ~ *Dr. John Przybylak, DC*, Chiropractic Rescue and the American Tragedy

Informal efforts are where the story begins. As downtown disappeared into piles of steel and ash on 9-11, New Yorkers reappeared and opened their hearts; Chiropractors hurried out of office shelters into sites of attack, delivering care.

Formalities were soon installed as Ground Zero declared a crime scene requiring the highest levels of security clearance. Now the New York Chiropractic Council had a groundbreaking crisis to resolve: how to get Chiropractic care on site. It was important the Council got this right. Chiropractic could easily be denied.

Dr. Ellen Coyne got it done. And for the first time in history, the American Red Cross worked with a Chiropractic organization, the New York Chiropractic Council, as part of disaster relief.

Dr. Coyne served as the Chiropractic Coordinator to the nationwide participants and provided licensing and malpractice credentialing to approximately 1,500 DC's. The Red Cross provided the next credential: the high security badge.

But did it matter? At a *crime scene*, what could Chiropractors do?

This:

> ...Over the course of eight months, close to two million tons of debris were removed from Ground Zero. The Chiropractors played an important role in this incredible feat. Your professional treatment of thousands of rescue workers helped all who were involved in the recovery efforts to persevere. You are among the many quiet heroes of September 11th whose contributions will not be forgotten.
> ~ *Raymond W. Kelly,* The Police Commissioner, City of New York, *Chiropractic Rescue and the American Tragedy*

The purpose of Chiropractors at Ground Zero was service. Over $1.5 million in Chiropractic care was donated, and DC's adjusted at up to five respite sites, twenty-four hours per day from September 28, 2001 to May 30, 2002, when all work at Ground Zero was completed.

The 1,500 Chiropractors who served could have stayed home, watched the news, and sighed, "Oh, that's too bad." But they knew care was needed. It took personal courage to go, the scene was pretty awful. They provided Chiropractic in the field, light in a place of darkness.

I was allowed to set a table up close to the rubble, but not without a hard hat and a mask. It was here I met Mark on my table. He came from California to volunteer and had been at the site since the beginning working as a specialized digger (mole). He told me he had been recovering human remains all week. I'll never forget his eyes and his smile when he handed me a cigar and told me it was for when he found a live one – which he promised he would do. His smile couldn't hide what his eyes revealed. I connected with a suffering, tired soul.
~ *Dr. Anthony Caliendo, DC, Chiropractic Rescue and the American Tragedy*

To create the story I researched every avenue: looked for photos, poured through stories appearing in the Chiropractic trades, and contacted Dr. John Przybylak, DC for a first hand account. I worked to get this out into the world, absolute, irreversible, and counted.

I wondered who would see it, what would happen, who would care?

My research discovered that Chiropractic's efforts were already noticed. A commentary by the Disaster Research Center, University of Delaware, *Rebel Food, Renegade Supplies: Convergence After the World Trade Center Attack* recognized Chiropractic for its collaboration with the Red Cross. They witnessed that Chiropractic produced no management issues and offered a specific skill that was useful, performing spinal adjustments.

Finally the article was completed and published, in the *Journal of Vertebral Subluxation Research (JVSR)*, on April 19, 2004: "Chiropractic Rescue and the American Tragedy: The Chiropractic Relief Efforts at Ground Zero," by Drs. John Przybylak and Madeline Behrendt, with photos contributed by Drs. Glenn Scarpelli and Gary Deutchman.

I created a press release, which the World Chiropractic Alliance (WCA), publishers of *JVSR*, posted on a leading newswire service for journalists, media professionals, P.R. firms, government agencies, research institutes, non-profits, and medical schools.

Again I wondered who will see it, what will happen, who will care?

People cared. The press release was ranked #1 on *Newswise Top Hits* report for June 2004 *MedNews* stories. It was the leader in number of hits, over medical press releases about electronic brains, memory loss, or calorie burning.

To all the Chiropractors who served at Ground Zero, thank you, your exceptional performance is the story. To all those serving in sites of disaster around the world – thank you, your story deserves to be told.

What if I told you there is a Chiropractic story more popular than news about real electronic brains, or medical stories from the Mayo Clinic and Harvard, is that something you might be interested in? Is that a story you'd like to create?

Could you? *Would* you? Do it.

Audiences want the Chiropractic story – tell yours.

> The most amazing thing was the gratitude that a fireman expressed. It was obvious that he had been at Ground Zero for days. He looked numb, fatigued and completely worn out. His spine was ready for any kindness that I could offer...he offered to pay for the service...Amazing...God bless people like this man.

~ *Dr. Andrew DeWitt, DC, Chiropractic Rescue and the American Tragedy*

Write it, film it, blog it, screen it.

Because for *Anything, Nothing, and Everything* - there is Chiropractic.

- **Do not be fooled by what is on the outside.**
- **Interference affects activity of function.**
- **When looking at statistics remember there is a person there.**
- **See the person.**
- **Life is motion, motion is life; life stops without motion.**
- **Be proud.**

Lessons In Being
Dr. Wanda Lee MacPhee

Dr. Sarah was confused and not just a little frustrated. She had been doing everything she thought she was supposed to in order to be a great Chiropractor. She went to a good school, very rarely missed a class, was skilled in her techniques, and serving patients. However, practice wasn't turning out the way she envisioned. Sure, patients came in and some even sent in others for care. However, it seemed many of them were not taking her recommendations seriously. So many missed the messages she was trying to share. She knew she could help them to really change the quality of their life.

Why didn't they get it?

Maybe it was her town. Maybe it was the specific location of the office. Maybe it was the economy. Maybe she didn't have a big enough sign. Maybe her *Yellow Pages* ad didn't attract enough attention. Maybe it was her staff.

"I don't know what I'm *not* doing," she thought. "I'm doing everything I was taught! I guess I just need to learn to do it better."

So Sarah looked for more things to do. She took technique seminars, marketing seminars and management seminars. She hired new staff, changed her office décor and lowered her fees. She kept more detailed statistics and bought more advertising. She stayed open later and started practice earlier.

The feelings of success were fleeting, with small improvements to her business, though not to the extent Sarah inwardly knew she was capable. Moreover, her message was not completely received by her patients. She was doing more and more, only to remain stuck. Nothing quieted the voice in Sarah's head saying "This is *not* it." Sarah was not fulfilled.

On so many levels, Sarah had a wonderful life. She was married, had children, and her family brought her great joy in many ways. Still, the lack of fulfillment persisted. Friends and colleagues could not understand Sarah's discontent.

They told her, "You have a wonderful practice. You have a great lifestyle and a wonderful balance. What more could you want? Why work any harder if you don't have to?"

"Maybe they are right," thought Sarah. "Maybe I am just being selfish. I have a wonderful life and I should spend my time enjoying it instead of looking for something more." So Sarah slipped into a life of complacency, not really content with all of life's demands; but life felt *good enough.*

Truly, good enough wasn't *really* good enough. Soon Sarah didn't even know why she was bothering to work in her practice anymore.

"What difference does it make if I even show up at the office?" Even conceiving that thought was uncomfortable. It was the kind of uncomfortable sitting in the pit of her stomach, waking her in the middle of the night, driving her to run and hide, just to stop thinking.

"What else can I do?" She thought. "I have done everything I think I *can* do, yet I am not feeling fulfilled."

And then she felt another kind of uncomfortable. This time though, it made her feel like something big was about to happen, something scary and exciting at the same time: like a breakthrough in the making. At the time she wasn't fully aware, but what she was about to do would make all the difference. Although uncomfortable, she was on course for an amazing self-discovery.

In her quest for something new, Sarah committed to yet another seminar, this one different from the rest. This one wasn't about *doing* different; it was about the *common denominator* in everything she had already been doing. It was a seminar about *Sarah*.

Sarah discovered it wasn't about doing more.
Sarah discovered it wasn't about doing it better.
Sarah discovered it wasn't about doing it differently.
Sarah discovered it has always been about *BEing*.
Sarah began a new journey.

Her discovery fueled her to further self-examination. It made her take deep breaths to open her mind and heart to new levels of understanding. She recognized she possessed the vision for a brighter reality, and that it was waiting for her to be ready for it, as if to unveil a maze of lessons waiting to be learned.

Exploring the new maze was a bit scary and often confusing, while also challenging and fun. Nonetheless, Sarah became fully engaged in playing the game of life with a refreshed and vital outlook. The sense of complacency that trapped her for so long was replaced by a sense of curiosity for transformation.

Sarah started her journey through the maze of lessons with taking lots of notes and creating key reminder cards for herself. Soon, she had a stack of cards she called "Lessons in *BEing*."

Lesson in *BEing* #1: GRATITUDE IS A STATE OF BEING

In her first discovery, Sarah recognized she wasn't fully *BEing* grateful. Despite appreciating the gifts she received in life and feeling fortunate to have wonderful children, a loving partner, family and friends, a nice practice, she knew there was a deeper level of gratitude yet to be appreciated.

Being grateful for the good things in life is easy. It's natural to appreciate elements of life that fit into your ideal model. But what about appreciating challenge and adversity? The deeper *BEing* of gratitude holds no judgment of good and bad, of wanted and unwanted. It is simply a true appreciation and thankfulness for what *is*, no matter the circumstance.

> Make sure you count your blessings. Those who are grateful for what they experience in life will have more to be grateful for.
> ~ *Dr. John Demartini*

Full gratitude truly is a state of being. *BEing* grateful is a choice to have faith that all is exactly as it is meant to be in at any given point. *BEing* grateful is a choice to accept, allowing and rejoicing in what *is*, regardless of what it looks or feels like in the moment.

Sarah found the first Lesson in *BEing* could transform her life. Gradually and over time, gratitude became a more natural reflex. Sarah's first breakthrough in choosing to see her world from within and choosing to be grateful for life in all its expressions resulted in becoming a better wife, mother, doctor, friend, daughter and sister. She could be grateful even for adversity, because she accepted it was a force creating her to grow.

Lesson In *BEing* #2: IT'S ALL GOOD

Sarah had the long-standing pattern of labeling people, places, things and events as good or bad. The sense of gratitude she discovered in her first Lesson In *BEing* was powerful, but it was so much easier to be in the state of gratitude when she felt something was "good" versus "bad."

That's when she found the second Lesson in *BEing:* it's all good.

BEing grateful is a choice to trust that no matter the apparent positive or negative of the current situation, all is perfect and all is well and unfolding exactly as it should. If *BEing* grateful for life applies to all people, places, situations and events – no matter the circumstance of the moment – then how can there be good and bad? If in the end, there will be a gift – even if hidden from view at first sight – must life not always be good?

> There are only two ways to live your life. One is as though nothing is a miracle. The other is as though everything is.
> ~ *Albert Einstein*

With recognizing all as good, Sarah empowered herself. The daily stresses and annoying challenges she had experienced from the outside world simply faded to the background. Adding to her first breakthrough to be grateful for all that is, she removed labels of good or bad to void judgment. Sarah felt a new level of inner peace. Everything began making more sense, and she grew into living an inside-out life full of gratitude and acceptance.

Her momentum built, yet she sensed there was still progress to be made.

Lesson in *BEing* #3: NOT ALL BELIEFS ARE REALITY

Sarah reached a new understanding of how her method of thinking profoundly impacted her level of daily happiness and sense of fulfillment. She acknowledged her former belief in labeling things good or bad created a block for being able to appreciate the Intelligence of the greater Universe around her. It was outside in rather than inside out and disempowered her. She set out to examine new ways of using her thoughts for empowerment.

To begin, she looked at old beliefs she *absorbed* over the years. Describing the beliefs as *absorbed* was the best way of admitting she didn't recall actually *deciding* to believe one thing or another. Somewhere along the way, an outside influence – well intentioned or not – implanted beliefs she thought to be reality, as if she had been viewing the world through distorted lenses. She took the liberty of changing her glasses!

> A belief is just a thought you keep thinking.
> ~ *Abraham-Hicks*

Sarah's beliefs surrounding love, happiness, expectations, activities, work, money, and success were brought into focus under her microscope. Writing down each subject, she defined her beliefs within. To her discontent, the activity of characterizing her beliefs affirmed there were far more beliefs creating less than desirable feelings. No wonder she was unable to reach the destination in life she originally set for herself, feeling unfulfilled. Her internal GPS was outdated and the road she was looking to travel did not exist in the map she was working with.

Well, if a belief was a thought you keep repeating, then what might happen if she starts *thinking* something else? Could it really be that easy?

The beliefs she had written down needed altering. She redefined the beliefs that did not serve her, and slightly tweaked or left alone the beliefs serving her well. Sarah's beliefs about herself, her children, her partner, her practice, her patients and others in her life evolved from rigid and often unrealistic, to allowing, accepting, and celebrating. The concept was simple, but the transition to adopting and applying new thoughts was a true test.

Frequently, she caught herself thinking old limiting beliefs. Some served her, but not others. When an old belief crept in, she consciously shifted her thinking to what she decided was her new belief.

When she caught herself thinking of something as a true belief, Sarah learned to re-examine it, question if it was indeed reality. She discovered some of the tools needed for a full transformation of her thinking in Byron Katie's book, *Loving What Is.*

The freedom to let go of concepts of what she previously perceived as absolute reality offered a complimentary understanding that there are as many realities as there are people to interpret a situation. Sarah freed herself of expectations, reactions, and judgments she unconsciously imposed upon herself and others.

Lesson in *BEing* #4: CREATE A GAME YOU CAN WIN

Throughout her practice as a Chiropractor, Sarah was conflicted. She loved serving people; she loved making a difference in their lives, but was also a Mommy and loved her children more than anything in the world. Though she believed she was a good Chiropractor and a good Mommy, there was still a sense of uneasiness about the two conflicting beliefs. Sarah reconsidered the rules she was living by.

In re-examining her definition of reality, she realized many rules and expectations she established for herself and others were incongruent or downright incompatible. No wonder she didn't feel she was making a difference: the rules and expectations did not promote one another; they were unattainable without having to make an exception for another rule.

Her expectations for being a Chiropractor were to be available for patients and not be away from the practice for too long. In her expectation, a *good* Chiropractor should have patients who understand how Chiropractic helps them to live better, should have a busy practice, and work many hours. She also held expectations about giving back to the profession and keeping up with the latest information and knowledge by attending continuing education classes and seminars. Because of this, Sarah attended many seminars. Yet she had difficulty in maximizing and enjoying the experience due to conflict with her expectations of her to *also* be a good Mommy.

Sarah's rules for being a Mommy told her she should be at home with her kids; she is supposed to attend events and parent-teacher interviews; she is supposed to bake cookies and make lunches in the kitchen; she is supposed to stay home and take care of the children if they became sick. Obviously, her beliefs were not aligning. How had this gone unnoticed until now?

> Placing the blame or judgment on someone else leaves you powerless to change your experience. Taking responsibility for your beliefs and judgments gives you the power to change them.
> ~ *Byron Katie*

Sarah had a new appreciation for the dilemmas created within her expectations. She could not be in two places at once, and the demands she placed upon herself with *shoulds* could never be fulfilled. Looking deeper, she recognized many of her expectations for her success and fulfillment were dependent upon other people. How much control did she really have over the scheduling of parent-teacher interview or seminars? The game could not be won without a change in her expectations.

"What if the new rules are more simple?" Thought Sarah. What if a Chiropractor did the best she could for each patient when she was present? What if it wasn't her job to make someone else healthy, but to simply do her best in the moment? What if her children were experiencing learning from many people in their lives and she was not their only provider? What if the rules were just about making time really count by *BEing* fully present with her children, her patients, her partner and the others in her life, rather than trying to do everything all at once? In the process of examination, she redefined the game she was playing.

Lesson in *BEing* #5: YOU CAN ONLY CONTROL YOU

Sarah tried to orchestrate life on her own terms. Not just her life, but also the lives of her children, husband, family, patients, and friends. With loving intentions, Sarah was doing everything she could think of to help, to guide, to assist, to teach, to instruct, and sometimes to convince other people. The frustration, she realized, came from the mistaken belief she had control over the outcome of the help, guidance and assistance she offered. When others did not respond the way she anticipated with her orchestration, she felt like a failure.

> The highest state of awareness is where you realize there's no separation between cause and effect, where your perceptions are the true causes and your reactions are the true effects of your life, where you are the cause of your own effect.
> ~ Dr. John Demartini

By releasing the need to have someone else act, think, feel or say anything in a way she expected, Sarah opened up the possibility of creating her own experience of life. Sarah began to see how all of the aspects of her *BEing* influenced her own level of fulfillment in life. No longer living in reaction to external sources, her way of *BEing* began shifting to focus inwardly. She discovered her vital authenticity with all the power she needed over her own experiences.

Lesson in *BEing* #6: THE POWER OF PURPOSE

Sarah has always prided herself on getting things done. She was an excellent *do-er*. She did it all, and if it didn't workout the way she planned, then she just did more of it and did it better. Previously, she spent much of her *doing-*

time focusing on unattainable outcomes independent from her control. Sarah fell into a trap of using action to create urgency, a feeling of value, and to fulfill her from the outside in.

In reviewing and rethinking her beliefs, her rules, and her behaviors, Sarah discovered *doing* was as unfulfilling as having incongruent expectations. Under her new realization of creating beliefs congruent with reality, she ascertained the belief that action does not equate to accomplishment. This discovery was pivotal for Sarah. Her lesson transcended from the emotional and theoretical into the day-to-day physical nature of life.

The *must do's* and the *should do's* and the *have to do's* were not fulfilling. Sarah did them because she could and should, but didn't share that sense of greater purpose for doing them. However, she loved *doing* things that created feelings of fulfillment, such as making a difference and contributed to others. This was *doing* with a purpose.

Delivered to a new perspective, she asked herself the greatest question, "Why?" Why she did what she did. When doing something unfulfilling, was there a different reason for doing it than when doing something fulfilling? The answer, an absolute "yes."

> The only reason we really pursue goals is to cause ourselves to expand and grow. Achieving goals by themselves will never make us happy in the long term; it's who you become, as you overcome the obstacles necessary to achieve your goals, that can give you the deepest and most long-lasting sense of fulfillment.
> ~ *Anthony Robbins*

Sarah took a long look at what she was doing in all the areas of her life. She looked at where she had fallen into a trap of *doing* based on her old rules and beliefs. After weeks and months of examining her choices and actions, Sarah began to naturally replace the things that were just busy

activities with purpose driven actions that quickly acceler-
ated not only her sense of accomplishment but also her level
of inner fulfillment.

Lesson in *BEing* #7: THERE IS NO "THERE"

Sarah had spent months unraveling these Lessons in *BE-
ing*. Just when she thought she was getting a handle on
things and had reached the end of her journey, another new
lesson seemed to appear. In fact, not only were there more
breakthroughs, but also the pace of change and inspiration
seemed to be accelerating.

Sarah was amazed! She had come such a long way from
where she started: she never had a better relationship with
her husband, children, family and friends...even strangers
seemed to want to be around her. Practice was not only fulfilling but fun and more and more people were attracted to
the great energy and peaceful sense of herself generated by
just *BEing*. Sarah felt she was the ultimate creator of her
wonderful life, and daily felt a deep sense of gratitude and
fulfillment. Sarah made it through and she was where she
always wanted to be.

Sarah decided she probably was finished with her journey, and it was time to bask in the reward of all of her hard
work. She tried to stop thinking of new ideas. She tried to
avoid books, audios, seminars and Internet sites that lead her
into more discoveries. Sarah started losing that sense of
purpose and fulfillment she had finally found.

"When am I going to get there?" Thought Sarah. "I have
spent so much time and energy discovering so much, surely I
have learned enough lessons to mastering myself and my
practice by now? Where are these feelings of discontent
coming from?"

Sarah turned back to the Lessons in *BEing* that had got-
ten her to her place of well-*BEing* and fulfillment. Sarah read
through her notes again and realized she was seeing the les-

sons and gifts in a new light and learning even more from the same lesson.

Sarah was not the same Sarah who made the first round of Lessons in *BEing*. From her new understanding of herself, appreciation for the miracles of the Universe, and sense of purpose, Sarah was reading the notes with new eyes and hearing the voices with new ears, gaining new insight. The new lessons she was learning were there all along, but waiting for her to be ready. And wouldn't the same be true the next time as well?

> You could not step twice into the same river, for other waters are ever flowing on to you.
> ~ *Heraclitus*

Sarah found the final breakthrough of her Lessons in *BEing*. In her past focus on *doing doing doing*, Sarah was always acting to get it done. At the end of an activity was a fleeting sense of accomplishment, brief but quite addicting. With Sarah's new discoveries of *BEing*, she applied the same rules to seeking the "there," meaning an end target was reached, a mission accomplished, a reward earned. But *BEing* didn't work that way.

That was the ultimate Lesson in *BEing* for Sarah. There is no "there." Life is not a destination and to stop the journey is to stop life itself. *BEing* is a process and an ongoing creation of who she is and who she is becoming. The joy is not only found in the journey...the joy is the journey itself.

For those of you reading, I am sure there are a few wondering if this is simply a retelling of my own story. Sarah certainly has many similarities to my life as a woman, mother, wife, daughter, sister, friend...and Chiropractor. But Sarah isn't me. Sarah is the combined story of so many wonderful women, friends, colleagues, students, and mentors – people I had the gift of sharing a piece of my journey with. I honor each of them for both their courage in *BEing* and their gifts to me along the way.

- **Move from excuses to accountability.**
- **Gratitude is a state of *BEing*.**
- **Our beliefs may not be others' reality.**
- **Create a game you can win.**
- **Power is in purpose.**

Once Upon A Time
Dr. Pat Gayman

Once upon a time a little girl was born who innately knew she was destined to be in the healing arts. She thought she would be doctor. What a blessing, her journey presented the wonderful world of vitalistic care known as Chiropractic.

When I was asked to participate in this publication I was both thrilled and honored. With almost fifty years of passion for Chiropractic and a life journey that included many different methods of practice and professional experiences, surely I could write something to help others with ease. I understand the purpose of this publication is to inspire, encourage and motivate women to fan their passion for Chiropractic, to persist in following the dream that took them to Chiropractic college in the first place, to have the courage to continue no matter the challenge and examples of ways to pick yourself up to stay on course. Writing is far more challenging than I expected. What stories do I choose to touch you? How can I reach out and hug you with words? So here goes.

My first encounter with Chiropractic was in a Laundromat. Talk about "You never know how far reaching something you may say or do will affect the lives of millions." In this case, I struck up a conversation with a woman who recently graduated from Palmer School of Chiropractic, the school's name at the time. She bubbled over with enthusiasm as she described how her new practice was growing with people whose health was changing from being adjusted.

When we met at her office she told me how the nervous system controls all functions of the body, passing messages through the spinal column and spinal nerves for the purpose of healing and maintaining the body. Immediately I wondered why I never heard of Chiropractic before. I suffered migraine headaches, for gosh sake, and nothing the medical profession had to offer touched them. The mechanics of Chiropractic and the way it honors the body's wisdom made sense to me right from its introduction. Three weeks after my first adjustment I knew I had found my life's path. It wasn't long before I was in college.

Those were the days I refer to as my 'good old days.' I learned so much and met such wonderful people from all over the world. During that time, one of my great experiences was being the Chiropractic Assistant (CA) in the office of the man who was also the Clinic Director at the school. I was a pretty good CA, but I didn't apply what I learned from that experience to my own practice. I'll clue you in with full details later on.

I loved learning the Science and Art of Chiropractic, although my passion for this great profession grew as I gained understanding of the Philosophy of Chiropractic. Upon graduation, I returned home to the Monterey Peninsula of California. One day while sitting on a rock on the gorgeous coast of the Pacific Ocean watching the waves crashing-in, hitting against the rocks and gracefully kissing the sandy beach before retreating, I felt an odd sensation. My body, my entire being stopped 'vibrating' – a release of the stress from the intensity of the college years. As I sat there, the warm sun sparkling off the water, watching the waves come in and go out, I was struck with a deep understanding of the meaning of Universal Intelligence in all things. The action of the waves coming in and going out gave me an awareness of tides rising and falling, tide pools dying and then being reborn again, teeming life in the ocean imprinted the truth and beauty of Chiropractic on my mind and in my heart. Later, it became common practice for me to recommend everyone to take time after graduating to find their 'rock' so they can integrate the profound truth of Chiropractic into their very being.

The analogy of a Chiropractic adjustment as being like turning up the dimmer switch on a light has always been one of my favorites, because truly Chiropractic illuminates the Light within. The Philosophy of Chiropractic begins with the Major Premise: "A Universal Intelligence is in all matter and continually gives to it all its properties and actions thus maintaining it in existence." Further, our Philosophy states there is Innate Intelligence in each of us that is part of this all-encompassing Intelligence. Yes, we have infinite Light within. Innate is always 100 percent and the Intelligence within the body is carried from the brain over the nervous system into every cell. That's where Chiropractic comes in.

So, what dims the light? Subluxations of the spine, causing interference with transmission of intelligent messages from the brain into the tissue cells. An easy example to illustrate to people everywhere is the Safety Pin Cycle: a closed safety pin has a complete cycle, where as an open safety pin has a broken cycle and is disconnected. Chiropractic keeps the connections within the nervous system functioning at full capacity.

A second 'light dimmer' is *stinkin' thinkin'*. Maybe you've heard the phrase "What you think about comes about." Our brains are hardwired with thoughts that have potential to either support us or narrow our possibilities. Neuroscience has shown we can create new habits of thought and weaken the old ones by changing our thinking. This is an important concept to aid you in life and can be taught to patients who may have fear about their health or are dealing with stress in unhealthy ways.

Chiropractic is balanced in its approach, as it includes philosophy as a foundation, science for understanding the body, and art for the skill of removing subluxations. Art is your technique when you have become unconsciously competent with it, and apply philosophy by an innate to innate connection with your patients. Remember, we are all connected at an energetic level (referring back to the Major Premise). You adjust, innate heals.

Renegades Among Us

Many of you reading this book were not even a glimmer in someone's eye when my Chiropractic life began. At the risk of being one of those silver seniors who talks about the good old days, I believe there is value in knowing some of the highlights of the choices and influences that brought our profession to this point in time. It has been said the value of history is to better understand the happenings of today.

Women have a colorful and interesting history, starting with the first class of fifteen students – three females at a time when women were not allowed into most medical schools. In 1904, Mabel Heath Palmer's graduation signaled the beginning of a strong women's influence on the profession. Dr. Mabel, known as "The First Lady of Chiropractic" was a model showing us it is possible to successfully wear the many roles of a woman *and* make a profound difference in the professional world.

In those days there were so many conflicting messages about the role of women. Women could not even vote at that time. Clear into the mid 20th Century, women for the most part did not give much consideration to actually owning a business to practice Chiropractic. Even Dr. Mabel said, "A woman's thorough knowledge of Chiropractic enables her to apply these governing Laws of Nature; I know of no better way in which a women can serve her family, her home, and her friends than by educating her in the Chiropractic profession." Notice there is no mention of actually practicing or serving her community. At that time, it was common for many women graduates to become assistants to their husband's practice.

There are those few dynamic women noted in our history to brave private practice, and some who paid a very high price for the right to practice. If you ever question your own passion for Chiropractic, imagine having your right to practice taken away from you. Some of the pioneers of our profession were willing to go to jail at a time when prisoner's rights were unknown. Imagine the cold, rat infested jails of old with surly guards willing to do who-knows-what to a female prisoner. Perhaps the worst of it would be the separation from your children and loved ones. Would you be able to practice without continued harassment? What would happen next?

Thanks to those who endured these hardships we don't have to fear for our licenses. Yet courage is still needed to stand up and tell the *truth*, without 'selling out' to the pain and musculoskeletal model of Chiropractic. Frankly, clarity in your message, commitment to Principles, and courage is what it takes to be hugely successful in practice.

Of my many mentors, two in particular stand out for me. Dr. Tina Murphy, from the Deep South, was one of the few women practicing the technique I chose to practice upon graduating – upper cervical technique. She was a true gentlewoman in every way, and taught me the power of gentle strength – sort of like a stream capable of eventually eroding obstacles in its way. At a terrible time in my life she loaned me some money, and said I was not to pay it back to her, rather I should give it to another woman who might be in need. From her I learned the beauty of 'pay it forward.'

Another of my mentors taught me persistence and determination in the face of adversity. I first met Dr. Rita Schroeder when I was on the Board of Regents of Pacific States Chiropractic College – later to become Life West. Two wonderful men founded the college. Their intention was to have a Principled college that also taught NUCCA, the upper cervical technique of my choice. The college was struggling financially and its President moved on to greener pastures. The Council of Chiropractic Education (CCE) dictates that for a college to exist and the student credits to count, there must be a President. The day the Board learned of the departure of the 'greener pastures' guy, someone turned to Rita and said, "Why don't you become acting President?" She may have been the most logical choice: because her mother had been an Administrator at another college at one point, or because she was part of a huge family of Chiropractors, or because she was married to a Chiropractor, or because her six children were (or became) Chiropractors and three of them were married to other DC's, or because she agreed to do it.

The presidential search that ultimately lead to the hiring of Dr. Gerard Clum took much longer than anticipated. During those many long months, Dr. Rita commuted 170 miles each way from her practice to the college every month and on other occasions as needed. She still had children at home; she endured an ugly divorce and still she maintained an active practice all in that same year. She was a tough lady in tough times and loved Chiropractic and her family. At the time of her passing there were more than seventy Chiropractors in the Schroeder-Molthen family. Talk about sharing the passion.

These are a few of the renegades who showed us the way!

It Really Was A Man's World

In spite of the early acceptance of women into Chiropractic schools, around the time I enrolled the percentage of women was around 5 percent. The percentage remained at that number for quite some time, gradually inching up to around 25 percent in the Eighties and Nineties; now in some schools 50 percent of the students are women. Unfortunately, there is still a higher attrition rate among women who leave or never even start practice. I have identified at least two reasons for this drop out rate for women; one is the decision to have a family and to stay at home to care for them, the other is distaste for and inadequacy at running a business. As a result, the percentage of women in the profession is nowhere near the number of women graduating.

Leave it to me to choose a male dominated profession in a world that still believed nice girls grew up, got married and had babies, rather than pursue a career of any kind. While at Palmer, and for a long time afterward, I was chosen to be the Secretary, rarely President or VP, of most organizations I chose to join. Women were seldom able to obtain a bank loan without a husband (or any male) to co-sign for them. My own Dad taught me I could do anything I set my mind to and encouraged me to be a doctor; but he also informed me I should stay home with my two kids.

Soon after I set up my first practice (stay tuned – there were more that followed), I decided to venture out and attend a Chamber of Commerce meeting. With great trepidation, I ventured forth into a world that was *not* Chiropractic for the first time since I actually became a Doctor. The very nice lady in charge of greeting new people made me feel very welcome.

I thought, "Okay, so this isn't so scary after all." The very first person she introduced me to was a man, the owner of a very popular local grocery store. He looked at me curiously (it may not have really been disdain as I imagined) and said with a bit of a sneer, "I've never met a lady bone-crusher be-fore." I was crushed. My newly acquired professional standing was crushed.

"Why are you even trying to do this technique? Women can never do this technique right anyway." That was the comment made by a man who conducted monthly work-shops to help us hone our NUCCA adjusting and analysis skills. One of my prize possessions is a letter he sent a few years later stating I had better adjusting and analysis skills than most men doing the work.

When CCE came along and continuing education became a requirement, seminars began to spring up all over and you guessed it: they were all taught by men. Women teachers in the colleges were also few and far between, so our education was, and much too often still is, focused from a male perspec-tive.

In all fairness, women were not doing much to neutralize the male dominant influence on the profession, even as more equality was happening in the 'outside' world. There have always been a few pioneering women who are models of what can be accomplished when one focuses on a desired outcome. For inspiration, I urge you to examine what is known of these women, because it was their passion for Chi-ropractic, determination, and courage that contributed greatly to maintaining Chiropractic as a separate and distinct profession. One of the best sources for information about these pioneers can be found in the wonderful book entitled *Chiropractic: An Illustrated History*, by Dennis Peterson, M.A. and Glenda Wiese, M.A.

The Road Less Traveled Without A Map

On my son's eighth birthday I opened the mailbox to find the long awaited, coveted license to practice Chiropractic. I was ready! In an act of naïve and foolish enthusiasm, I had already leased an office space. Then, the 'nice' equipment man came along. Since I was married and my husband was willing to co-sign on a lease, I was set up with nothing but the finest equipment to fill every bit of the overly large space I leased. I had just about enough equipment to run two practices.

I was so passionate about Chiropractic I was certain people would line up to receive the wonderful gift of Chiropractic. So it never crossed my mind to read all of the fine print of the equipment lease, spelling-out what happened if the leasor could not make the required payments. I was so sure it would never be a problem. The best part, the payment was kind of low for the first two years, and then it went up a whole bunch. I was certain I would have plenty of money by the time the price increased.

I was successful in that practice, in the way of attracting lots of patients. There was one little glitch though; I sort of forgot to talk to them about my fees that were a whopping three dollars after the initial exam and x-rays. Each time a new patient came in, I became so excited; however, I was afraid if I talked about money they wouldn't want to come back. It took a long time before I learned the concept of value exchange.

Two years passed and it started getting ugly. No amount of negotiating changed the fact that he wanted his big payments starting immediately. The saddest part was I had a relatively large amount of money in accounts receivable, money due to me for service I had rendered but waited too long to try to collect. Some lessons are harder than others. Finally I was forced to file bankruptcy. I was sure my precious Chiropractic career was over.

Fortunately, I have always been very determined and persistent. So even in the face of this failure I could not imagine not following my path by helping people through Chiropractic. After a short time of licking my wounds, I opened another practice in a remote little community way out of town. This time I did it the way I should have opened the first one.

In a small open space, I had an adjusting table with a screen separating it from a filing cabinet, a desk and a chair. It was charming and I was following my bliss. I befriended the MD across the street with the idea that he would take my x-rays for me, only to find out that the AMA prohibited any professional interactions with Chiropractors! Thank you Dr. Wilkes for changing that fact!

Each step of the way was like flying without a net. I did not know a female colleague to turn to for guidance or support. One of my classmates was working as an associate, and the other was having babies and running her husband's office. Practice managers had not yet come into the scene. I only knew I was meant to practice and to make myself available to help people. My family loved living in the country and my practice was growing slowly.

The privilege of watching one miracle after another touched my heart and motivated me to continue. Healing occurs in the most wonderful ways. A story that has stayed with me over all the years involves a common occurrence in Chiropractic offices, and is a reminder of how one adjustment can change a person's life.

A woman in her mid-thirties and about midway through pregnancy with her first baby came into my office as a patient. It was a time when delivering a baby was considered to be the domain of medical doctors and was controlled in the way he prescribed, having nothing to do with the wishes of the parents (even more extreme than it is today). Still, she was determined to go through pregnancy and delivery the *old-fashioned way.* She took great care of her self, ate the right foods, exercised, got adjusted and nurtured her unborn baby in every way possible. She absolutely glowed with joy.

After the delivery I did not hear from her for about six weeks. One Friday afternoon, she came dragging into my office, looking like she aged at least ten years. She was drawn and haggard, and there was no light in her eyes. Her little bundle of joy had been miserable and caused misery during most of his short life. No one slept. He cried and his parents tried everything to comfort him. They cried but still he did not stop crying. He had colic. Somehow, I had not educated her on the importance of having the baby and she checked after the birth.

I took the little 'cry baby,' adjusted him and his Mom, and sent them home. Sunday morning I got a call. When I answered, the woman on the line was crying, and when she identified herself, my heart nearly stopped. My worst fear: an adjustment gone wrong and something horrible happened to the baby. But, no. Her tears were of joy, of relief, and the voice I heard was from a woman whose baby just slept through the night.

Just as I was settling in with this small, part-time practice a fantastic opportunity opened up to me. One of my mentors, Dr. George E. Anderson offered me a part-time position as an associate. Associate positions were not common in those days, so I was thrilled. Even though the practices were in separate towns, I was able to work with him a couple of days a week and still keep my sweet little office running. Dr. Anderson was a white haired, distinguished looking gentleman whose main interest in hiring me was in seeing how people responded to a woman in practice. I became very proficient at reading x-rays and using the neurocalometer for thermal scans of the cervical region. However, the only time I was allowed to adjust was when Dr. Anderson was out of the office. After all, I was 'just a girl,' how could I possibly be a

competent doctor? It was only through Dr. Anderson's as-
surances that people ever agreed to have me adjust them. I
am forever grateful to him for his faith in me.

So, in less than five years I had a full time practice, went
bankrupt, had a part-time practice and became an associate.
By the way I also got divorced and remarried. *Life* just keeps
on happening.

Wonder-Woman Syndrome

Wonder-Woman, super—mom—doctor—businesswoman—
community leader—wife, no problem. Just like *Wonder-
Woman*, I acted like I had super powers and figured *some day*
I would slow down and take time to care for myself. *Hint*: In
case any of you belong to the *Wonder-Woman* species, this is
a *very important* point: *some day* never comes unless you
initiate it.

A wonderful patient introduced me to her son, the man
and love of my life. I know it sounds corny, but it was truly
love at first sight. It wasn't long before we decided to get
married. There was just a moment's hesitation, as I contemplated what it would be like to take on *five more children*!
Yes, my honey had five children who needed a mother to care
for them. So I did, and still do. Talk about flying without a net.
With two children it was fun to experience new things as
they grew, meshing my schedule with theirs' with relative
ease. Now there would be seven children ranging in age from
seven to fourteen-years-old. It was like having two sets of
twins plus three.

The following years were challenging, wonderful and awful all at the same time. We integrated the families – my two
children with his five and moved away from the watchful
eyes of our extended families. I took a couple of years off to
help this happen. These were the years I refer to as the

'bleacher-butt' years. It made sense to me to get that little mob of children involved in extra-curricular activities, ranging from Little League to swim team to rodeo to cheerleading and more. I was there in the stands.

Finally, I felt the time was right to find an office where I could practice as an independent contractor. I quickly had a good base of patients from the parents I met in the bleachers and people from my *Avon* territory. I practiced part-time so I could be on the bleachers and available after school. It was important to both of us for our children to develop a decent work ethic and to know the satisfaction of a job well done. I made sure they had plenty of chores and responsibilities around the house and garden so they could learn skills that would serve them as adults. Actually, I am grateful, during those years we did not have the financial resources to shower the kids with every little thing their heart desired. As a result, they learned independence and how to work for what you want in life. They have become wonderful, self-sufficient adults and that is a joy to me.

About the *Wonder-Woman* Syndrome: I was sure I could do it all, and even bake all the family bread so they would eat truly healthy food, and so on. Enough already! The lesson I had to learn was to say *no*. I was trying to be all things to all people and not leaving enough for myself: emotionally, spiritually, or physically. That never works. It has taken many, many years for me to really *own* that lesson.

The home that was once under siege by five teenagers living there at once finally started emptying, as one kid after another began to graduate from High School and embarked on their own life's journey.

Joy On The Journey

After being an independent contractor, it was time for me to establish my own practice on a full-time basis. It was incredible – wonderful and very challenging. These were the golden years of insurance for Chiropractic, and proper codes and billing procedures were established. We billed and they paid. Nice!

They were golden years for me in many ways, as I experienced the miraculous changes that regularly occurred for people who had no interference between brain and body, those whose nervous systems were functioning at full capacity and whose Innate Intelligence could heal their bodies naturally without drugs or surgery. I was witness to much irrefutable evidence that the body is a self-healing mechanism as long as there is no interference to the system controlling it. Adjustments resulting in relief from low back pain or migraine headaches may not be as dramatic as the healing experienced by a patient whose hearing is restored, or the child handicapped from severe asthmas who becomes the track star in high school; but, dramatic or not, if you are the one with the back pain or the headache, the relief from an adjustment can be life changing. I can testify to that because I had suffered from migraine headaches until I was blessed with a Chiropractic adjustment.

Many might deem one particular experience a true miracle. A fifty-year-old man diagnosed with amyotrophic lateral sclerosis (ALS/Lou Gehrig's disease) came to me for care. He was braced from head to foot, with a cervical collar, thoracic support and braces on both legs, and walked with forearm crutches. He was a very sick man with what is considered an incurable disease.

While he was under my care, I learned a whole bunch about the emotional interactions occurring between doctor and patient. I didn't ever accept the common idea of his condition being an incurable disease, and frankly I became very attached to getting rid of the symptoms – even though I knew my only real job was to remove subluxations to restore communication between his brain and his body. As I became more involved with advising him on lifestyle changes, including eliminating the addictive pain medication he was taking, I learned he was estranged from his family. A lonely and very sick man, I offered him compassion and nurturing. Then something terrible happened – he developed a crush on me! He was fifteen hundred miles away from the home where he was not really welcomed. There were no other upper cervical practitioners locally. I felt I couldn't really dismiss him as a patient. This was a scary time, but finally he was convinced it really wasn't me but the care he was receiving that infatuated him. I kept adjusting him.

It took twenty-one and a half years before he walked across the tarmac to get on a plane to take him home. He had been reunited with his family and we were all filled with gratitude and awe at the transformation in his health. He was free of all braces except for one brace on his leg for the footdrop, his only remaining symptom. He walked without crutches and stood upright to his full six foot, seven inches. In all aspects this was a miracle healing.

Over the years, I learned about running a business like a business through the school of hard knocks. Experiences in my first solo practice, as an associate, as an Independent Contractor and finally back to solo, and then onto a multidisciplinary clinic all combined into the creation of Gayman Chiropractic and Wellness Resource Center, one of the top 2 percent of offices in the nation. One of the things I learned is that the people you choose to be part of your team are critical to your success. Include a good attorney on your team. A good front desk person or office manager can be an angel in your life, but a bad front desk person can bring disaster.

Finally I got it right. The business was run like a business, and I had an angel as an office manager. Life was good, business was booming and people were being served!

My World Began To Shake

Yes, I live in California, but no, the shaking was not from an earthquake. Instead, it was from events beginning on the first day in January, starting with a ruptured appendix. Less than a month later my mother died. Then in March, my husband and I decided to take a little road trip to celebrate our anniversary, and a drunken diver hit our car; it spun around and fell backwards over a fifty-foot ravine. A huge boulder stopped our car before landing in the river below. The ER doc was very concerned, and carefully stitched the gash over my eye so I would not grow old with a scar. And, oh by the way, he also said I had three compression fractures and a whiplash. Clearly orthopedics was not his strong suit. All I could think of was I had to get back to the office. I had been out of the office most of the month of January and part of February. My practice dropped in half, and I had a staff to take care of and patients who might be losing patience. At my insistence, the ER doc said I could only leave the hospital if I could walk out. Of course I could walk out: I was in shock and determined. The pain didn't really set in until a few hours later.

My true determination and persistence took over. Instead of crawling into a fetal position and feeling very, very sorry for myself (well okay, admittedly I did spend a little while sad and angry), I looked at my options and started making changes.

Instead of cutting back I decided to expand. I put all of the lessons of business I had learned to work, took inventory of my own skills and talents, and set out to reverse my damaged financial situation. I couldn't adjust, so I hired an associate. I stayed involved so the patients did not feel deserted and the practice began to recover.

Community activities took a great deal of my time. I showed up, kept my commitments, demonstrated I could be trusted. The inevitable outcome was that when they thought of Chiropractic, they thought of me. Gayman Chiropractic and Wellness Resource Center became the *go to* place in town. With complementary practitioners joining our team as independent contractors, our services continued to grow. It was a lively place, and thanks to my *angel* office manager it ran well.

The next few years were incredible. I started speaking at the Parker Seminars on a regular basis and eventually was traveling to speak at other associations. I received awards and accolades professionally and within the community. I met the *movers and shakers* in our profession and developed fabulous and lasting friendships. A great honor was bestowed upon me when I was asked to join the Royal Chiropractic Knights of the Round Table: an invitation-only group of powerful, dynamic, successful women. Attending Seminars and being involved in many ways in the profession helped fan my passion for the power of a Chiropractic adjustment and helped me stay current with the latest information available to practice.

Finally all the travel and the challenge of maintaining a large office took a toll on me. So, I decided to sell my practice to my associate. After the sale, I found myself back in part time practice in a small office. This arrangement had been spelled out in our sales agreement.

My marriage had become quite shaky, as well. My husband worked out of town all week while I often traveled on the weekends – not a good recipe for a strong marriage. After much deliberation, we decided being together was important enough for one of us to make a change.

The Road Takes A Turn

Call it destiny, if you will, but my decision to move to the San Francisco Bay area resulted in an unexpected path opening up: a path giving me yet another opportunity to be a part of our great profession. Not long after I moved, I heard Life West was looking for someone to teach an Office Procedures class for three hours a week. Even though I had no formal teaching experience, I figured that since I had experienced all types of practice models and done it wrong and done it right, surely I could impart some wisdom to help students.

To my great surprise and delight, Dr. Clum remembered I was on the Search Committee that hired him. I returned to an institution I cared a great deal about. My experience there was colorful, to say the least. Sometimes it was incredibly fulfilling and sometimes I wondered what in the world was happening?

The very next term after I started teaching the three hour class, I found myself an Administrator: Chair of the Division of Chiropractic Sciences. Talk about on the job training. I oversaw the Technique and Philosophy Departments. It was quite an adventure. Academia was a whole new world and I had to remember I could not forge ahead as if it were my own practice. After I unintentionally offended some of the faculty and other Administrators, I realized I had to learn there is certain protocol to be followed when you are part of a larger organization. As I taught students, they also taught me. I loved teaching Philosophy and being a part of helping people who were making Chiropractic their career, their life.

Then, I was promoted to Dean of Clinics. I was excited because I honestly thought I would be able to be more hands-on with the Interns and share some of my experience with patients. The reality of the position was different than I thought: too much administration, meetings, budgets, discipline and disgruntled faculty. I worked hard but I missed the fulfillment of directly helping people.

Remember my discussion about the *Wonder-Woman* Syndrome? It took over again, only in different form. I thought I could do it all and get around to taking care of myself later. One night I had a dream I was puzzling over while driving to the clinic. Innate *spoke* clearly, saying it was time to leave Life West. So I did.

Joy On The Journey

I am so grateful for the amazing skills I developed from being at the college. I know so much more about systems and budgets, procedures and protocol, hiring and training the right people, and overseeing an enormous practice (the Clinic) with three hundred associates (interns), sixty or so team members (faculty and staff). I felt more than qualified to step out as a Practice Coach.

To my delight, last year I was asked to return to Life West once again. This time I act as a consultant, going once or twice a term to the College to conduct Customer Service training for the Health Center Staff and Marketing for the Interns and Faculty. I feel truly blessed. Oh, by the way I also maintain a small part-time practice. I just couldn't keep my hands to myself any longer.

Bill Esteb, one of the premier communicators in our profession, once said to me, "Pat, you might as well grasp the fact that you are seen by many as the *Chiro* Mom." I decided to use that perception to fulfill my own purpose of helping people successfully live their dream. I know life has to have balance in it. To be truly authentic with patients you have to overcome limiting beliefs, taking your own counsel. Perfection will elude you but excellence, fulfillment and joy need not.

Back when I enrolled as a student, one of the epigrams on the walls at Palmer said, "Enter to learn, go forth to serve." I hope you continue learning bits of wisdom to make your journey easier and fulfilling. Let Universal Intelligence be your guide. Let your knowledge of Chiropractic guide the path of your service.

- **Turn up the dimmer switch.**
- **Be a renegade.**
- **Define your own world.**
- **School of hard knocks: have back up.**
- **We experience times when life is challenging, wonderful, and awful at the same time.**
- **Make your own joy along the journey.**

We Live The Life We Imagine
Dr. Jennifer Barham-Floreani

When we consider the special qualities that healers and health practitioners can offer the world, many come to mind, such as selflessness, intuition, and empathy. These beautiful qualities are found in both men and women, yet are often associated with women. Some say women take more time to consider and heal their own personal history, create a deeper awareness of themselves, and are more willing to look at their unconscious attitudes.

At the same time, I can think of many men in my life who exude the so-called *feminine* qualities and continue to teach me about the processes of self-healing. Therefore, as I begin this chapter, I am reminded it is futile to try to reduce anyone or any gender to a checklist. As a mother of four boys, I would rather nurture the vision of moving towards an age of clarity and understanding, a time of camaraderie between genders and peoples that will better unite us. While there may be human traits that are more common to women than men and vice versa, may we always remember to celebrate the learning that comes with the varied stages of life, and to celebrate the gift of human potential within us all.

Humble Beginnings

Being able to inspire a family to move towards a Chiropractic wellness lifestyle requires a voice of 'authenticity and certainty.' Finding this voice takes time, even when you are lucky enough to be born into a family of Chiropractors. I literally grew up in a home practice. My mother was my father's receptionist, and as the youngest of six children (with everyone else otherwise occupied with school or university), my role was to help my mother by leading the patients into cubicles where they would wait for my father to call them through to an adjusting room.

Despite this early exposure to Chiropractic, I learned the hard way that Chiropractic can be tricky to explain. I was only three years old when I was first called upon to describe my father's profession. My parents had entered me into a children's beauty pageant, an event that was held in a large department store, hosted by a well-known celebrity, and televised across our state. I found myself on the center stage for the award ceremony, my hair in ringlets, wearing a pink dress and shiny shoes. With cameras rolling and all eyes on me, the host introduced the segment and then turned to me with the microphone and said, "This is a very exciting day, Jennifer. Who are you here with, sweetheart?"

I replied, "Mummy. My Daddy is at work, he's a Chiropractor."

Surprised that such a small child was far from shy, the host smiled at the crowd and asked me again, "What is he, sweetheart?"

"A Chiropractor!" I yelled.

"Well that's a big word. Do you know what that means, Jennifer?"

"Yes."

"Well, tell us honey, what does a Chiropractor do?"

"It means he makes the ladies take their clothes off and he pulls their legs!"

One can imagine my parents' horror! At the time my quiet, unassuming father, having graduated only a few years previous and formally a radiographer, was in the habit of gowning female clients and asking men to remove their shirts before he adjusted them. This was a habit he quickly dropped after his daughter's stage-show performance. Needless to say, the incident presented a steep learning curve for the whole family and my Chiropractic education instantly became a high priority for my parents.

My father went on to inspire five of his six children and many of his grandchildren to become Chiropractors. I married a Chiropractor and my husband's family now has five Chiropractors in its ranks as well. With such a dynasty surrounding us, I can only hope we are fortunate to avoid a repeat public blunder with our own children. (Note to self: educate children on how to communicate Chiropractic from the moment they can speak or risk frightful public humiliation.)

Knowing Who You Are

Having personally watched from a young age the way babies, children and adults respond to Chiropractic, I am blessed to have acquired a 'certainty' about my health – a certainty I notice is often lacking in my peers. In an effort to bridge this gap, I became passionate about instilling all children with health confidence – not just those fortunate to grow up in our profession. I knew I wanted to play a role in empowering parents to raise healthy, *well adjusted* children.

With this in mind, when my husband and I bought our first practice, we set about transforming aspects of the business, such as its fee structure and scheduling system, to suit our own personal values and integrity. This was a critical time for us to ask ourselves:

- ♦ What types of care do we wish to offer?
- ♦ What types of clients do we wish to attract?
- ♦ How would we like our practice (and Chiropractic) to be viewed by our community?

At this time, most Chiropractors were in the habit of scheduling clients on a monthly maintenance basis. But I was uncomfortable with this style of care because I had always had my nervous system checked weekly. 'Wellness care programs' were mostly unheard of then, with the focus being mainly on crisis care, preventative care, and maintenance care. Yet we decided to add a set of more affordable fee structures that would allow families to include Chiropractic in their weekly health program, and to embrace true wellness lifestyles.

Because this fee structure hadn't been trialed, many of our friends and family were anxious about our decision to keep some of our prices so low. Yet it proved very popular, as we discovered a large group of clients who wanted to invest in proactive health.

As always, when we take action from a heart level rather than a financial level, the rewards are plentiful. Sometimes these actions take courage. It is easy to embrace the latest trend or promotional tool in an attempt to build business but in order to achieve longevity and fulfillment in a practice, we need to first define our higher ideals so that any protocols or programs implemented are congruent with who we are. A lack of authenticity is palpable to everyone around us.

> Not understanding yourself is not understanding the truth.
> ~ SOEN-SA

Many, many times in my life I have been compelled to consider: *What is my truth? What do I value? Am I being true to those values and who I am?*

We can all fall victim to believing we need to live by another's standards, yet one thing I have learned: life can be a beautiful blend of simplicity and richness when we live with a congruent heart. Be it in the sphere of work, parenting, or relationships, it means making choices that fuel our soul and feel right with every inch of our body.

This ideal is tested continually in the modern world where few of us are immune to the struggle of finding a work-life balance. And here it would seem that Mother Nature has thrown women a few extra curve balls. Women who love their careers and yet want to have children often find it tricky to know when to conceive, when to return to work, and how many hours are needed to still offer 'great service' to clients – not to mention running a business and a household to boot!

Irrespective of whether we have children or not, unless we define how we want to live our lives, it can be very easy to lose sight of who we are along the way. I believe if we commit a portion of our day to visualizing the life we desire in our hearts and minds first – as a priority above any other action – then we will meet success beyond our wildest dreams. Sometimes we try to create the life we want by working harder, acquiring more things, accumulating more money, or demanding things of others. We become so caught up in the *doing* we forget the power of staying in gratitude for the moment at hand, and the power of being *certain* we are in fact attracting our heart's desires. Certainty is extremely compelling to the Universe.

While "reality is an illusion—albeit a persistent one," as Albert Einstein once said, it is worthwhile to remind ourselves every day that we are the creative force in our life.

The Wisdom Of Experience

I believe families (be they traditional, extended, single parent or mixed families) are the core fabric of society. As such, I am extremely passionate about helping parents to navigate and strengthen their family's health outcomes, and my vision has always been to do so via improving parents' health literacy.

However, there was certainly a time in my life when my upbringing fuelled a degree of self-righteousness about the health choices parents sometimes make. As a new graduate and prior to having my own children, there were times I had to hide my exasperation as parents implemented decisions that seemed antagonistic to the holistic health ideals I tried steering them towards. Outwardly I respected their choices, but I had difficulty understanding them. Sometimes when we are passionate about things we are guilty of losing perspective.

Since then, life has thrown me numerous experiences that have allowed me to better gauge and appreciate the needs of today's parents, and to conceive of more insightful methods of inspiring them to learn about health. What I soon realized is that to have far reaching impact, it is not so much knowledge that is important, but our character and our attitude that counts. We can teach by example only when we ourselves are willing to be taught and when we have gained a deeper sense of humility that only life experience can bring. In comparison to those early years, the empathy and rapport I now have with parents is beautifully gratifying.

I believe the challenges we experience in life help us to reveal greater and greater versions of ourselves. Perhaps we discover some of our highest qualities only in tough times and darker moments, for when life is blissful we may not need to be as resourceful.

Our first birth still feels like a wonderful slap from Mother Nature. In my naivety and youth, I was certain I would have a straightforward, natural childbirth. I was an extremely capable woman – in fact, painfully so. I liked to be in control of all aspects of my life, and I viewed childbirth as merely a 'mind over matter' task, a worthy but 'manageable' conquest.

Yet life decided it was time to take me on a journey into the raw depths of true self-awareness. What was meant to be a quick, natural birth, free from intervention in a birth centre, became a thirty-six-hour hospital ordeal. Due to a combination of nervousness and pain, I managed to vomit with almost every contraction until we reached a point where I was completely dehydrated and our baby had turned posterior, extending his head backwards. Our waters were artificially broken, to no avail, and I remember lying in the hospital bed with tubes everywhere – an epidural, catheter and drip – wondering how on earth we ended up like this.

We had prepared so well and worked so hard. What had happened? I turned to my husband Simon who was sitting beside me; he looked pale and exhausted. He was holding my hand and I remember saying to him, "Life is such a great leveler, isn't it?"

After we had finally delivered our baby – dislocating my pubis (the joint at the front of my pelvis) in the process – I realized this experience had taught me to quiet my mind and to trust and listen to Spirit or Source. As it was once said, "You can be born with ability, you can acquire knowledge, you can develop skill, but wisdom comes from God."

Living Wholeheartedly

In the course of a lifetime we never know which events are going to support or teach us the most. Our second birth, in the comfort of our own home, was a beautiful, moment-to-moment lesson in surrendering, while our third birth was possibly the making of who I am today. Our baby, Abe, died in utero at twenty-eight weeks and we decided to deliver him without pain-relief, allowing me the opportunity to be fully present to my physical and emotional grieving. Experiencing the excruciating pain of bringing our son into the world, all the while knowing he had already died, certainly molded who I am today. Holding Abe in my arms and looking at him in awe for his external perfection, the concept of the 'frailty of life' took on new meaning. I still have no idea how we managed to leave him lying in his hospital crib and walk away. To this day that vision grips my heart so deeply that my knees still weaken. I am in awe of those who have experienced

enced greater loss than I and have managed to move forward, or of those families whose lives ebb and flow around a
child who has special needs. I have heartfelt respect for those
who embrace such challenges.

A week after delivering Abe, as I lay in bed, lost in a
world of grief, my body was overcome with infection. The
deep, deep longing I had in my heart to be able to hold my
child again was replaced by a deep aching in my joints, even
as I felt completely alienated from my physical body. I remember, as I was being prepped for a post-birth curette, a
voice deep within me exclaiming, "Enough!" It was time to
own my lesson in loss.

It has been said that the best way to maintain a memory
of a loved one is to carry on the wishes of that person. While
my journey of carrying Abe was brief, instinctively I knew his
life was a reminder for me to live wholeheartedly. Choosing
to do so is a decision. It is also a courageous pursuit. To live
wholeheartedly is a vision that calls me to action each day.

I experienced five births in all. The fourth was a lesson
again in learning to trust Mother Nature after such a recent
loss, while our fifth was a profoundly beautiful bonding experience for our family. Our births have allowed me to gain
tremendous knowledge in the parenting arena, and during
this procreative stage of our life, my husband and I also
birthed our holistic parenting book, "Well Adjusted Babies,"
an extraordinary success. Through this book, I have been
given an opportunity to connect with families across the
globe. As David Hawkins aptly put it, "We change the world
not by what we say or do but as a consequence of what we
become."

We Live The Life We Imagine

Over the years, my husband and I have been blessed to work
with many new graduates, and we found they have a com-

mon yearning to learn the secrets of building a successful practice.

When we look at the Principles involved, it quickly becomes obvious there is no separation between our inner and outer selves. Thus, when we develop ourselves, we develop our business as a byproduct.

While there are many skills and success Principles worthy of writing about, here are some of the essential insights we gathered over the years and continue to remind our selves of. They are simple commitments to self that help us live life more purposefully.

Essential insights:
1. **First we form habits; then they form us**. The rituals we create each day dictate the outcomes in our lives. This includes prioritizing time to stay motivated and inspired, and committing to habits that feed our mind and soul. It is imperative to invest in 'brain software' – reading inspiring books, listening to motivational speakers, attending personal development seminars, meditating, or visualizing. Self respect begins in our minds first.
2. **We are the company we keep.** Try to spend more time with people who inspire us to be joyous and to grow, and less time with people who have negative or judgmental outlooks.
3. **Hold a clear vision.** The clearer our vision of the life we desire, the quicker we manifest that life; the foggier our vision, the longer and more arduous the process of manifestation becomes. To hold our vision is to have faith in our Universe, which is endlessly bountiful and abundant.
4. **Pay strict attention to our thoughts.** When we learn to master our thoughts and quiet the ego, we accelerate the manifestation process. Every day I set myself the challenge of listening to the background

commentary in my mind and assessing if I am envisaging a grand future or instead wasting precious time and energy on worry, regret or self-criticism. I regularly check my internal dialogue to see if I am negating or empowering myself.

5. **Maintain a learning attitude**. We can accelerate our personal growth by consistently asking for feedback, transforming defensiveness, and maintaining a learning attitude. Most often defensiveness is driven by fear. If we can laugh at their own mistakes, and value the gift of self-awareness and self-renewal, we will find unexpected happiness. It is liberating to accept that we don't have all the answers.

6. **Stay in gratitude**. Being grateful for this life keeps our ego in check. Making time to give thanks is the quickest cure for 'stinking thinking'. It gives us energy, it's contagious, and it's deeply attractive. Life is much more rewarding when we celebrate the small successes as well as the large, and I like to remind myself to practice gratitude especially when I don't feel like it and with those whom I am struggling to appreciate.

7. **Be authentic**. Successful people live with integrity. They walk their talk, they speak their truth, and they keep promises to themselves and to others. This often requires courage. For example, new graduates might be tempted to over-promise results to their clients; however, it is better to commit to exemplary care rather then specific results or time frames. We don't always know what stressors are influencing people, nor can we predict their health outcomes. Let's be honest, and let's also admit when we don't know something or when we are wrong.

8. **Be responsible.** It is easy to be governed by our moods but there is great power in realizing we can control them. Rather than habitually responding in a

particular way to a person or a stressful situation, there is always a moment in time when we can consciously choose how we respond. Moods are contagious and have a ripple effect, so choosing consciously gives us a greater chance for happiness.

9. **Be present.** Staying present to yourself and others requires you to drop the internal dialogue and focus only on what is happening right now. *Thinking* is concerned with the past and the future, whereas *being* is about the now. Because 99 percent of your so-called problems do not exist in the now, by simply being present you can live a more authentic, creative and fearless life.

10. **Seek to understand, be empathic**. Giving someone your full attention is one of the greatest gifts you can offer. Through active listening we are better able to understand another person's rationale or viewpoint. This requires us to stay present and to stop presuming what their needs might be, or judging them for something we think is wrong. This is sometimes hard to do with loved ones or with people with whom we have conflicts, but if we start each day afresh and we consciously make the effort, we will find that we cannot judge and understand a person at the same time.

11. **Keep an abundant attitude**. Decide to consistently challenge your scarcity mentality and live with an abundant attitude instead. Know that there is enough for everyone and be happy for the success of others. Look for the good things in your life and celebrate those.

12. **Be a team player**. When living or working with others, keep in mind how your attitude is affecting them. Choose to limit complaints and criticisms, and be solution-oriented instead. Live with a strong spirit of co-operation and focus on mutual benefit.

13. **Be available.** Believe in the potential of people. Take a genuine interest in other peoples' lives, for there is great learning to be had when we are less self-absorbed. When we realize that the greatest success we'll know is by helping others succeed and grow, then our 'big love' attitude brings all the gifts of the Universe within reach.

14. **Give more than is needed.** When we choose to go the extra mile, giving away our time, expertise, money or things with no expectation of return, we are affirming our faith in love. True generosity is an act of love and an act of letting go. All that we have in this life is a borrowed gift meant to be passed on.

Be Available For Your Clients

I can clearly remember a newborn baby named Holly. I met her within the first few months of starting our practice. Holly was just three days old and she screamed nonstop while her mother tried to explain that her baby daughter had barely slept or fed since being born, and had been continually crying.

She was clearly unable to attach to the breast and the hospital staff had suggested that Holly's parents start using a formula.

I remember looking at this mother, and then at the grandmother who had come along to offer assistance, and then again to distressed little Holly. She had bruises along the right side of her face and down her neck, and when she cried, I could see that her tongue was also black with bruising. I took the mother's hand and asked, "Tell me about her birth."

Holly had been born with the use of forceps after the second stage of labor had been deemed excessively long. At no point had Holly's heart rate altered, but the doctors recommended assistance during the crowning stage. These same doctors later told Holly's parents not to be alarmed by her bruises, as sometimes this is an unfortunate but necessary complication; they said the bruises should subside in a few days.

What no one realized was that the forceps had dislocated Holly's jaw, which therefore affected her ability to open her mouth and breastfeed successfully. Not only was this little baby extremely hungry, she was also in excruciating pain.

It was wonderfully fulfilling to work with Holly intensively over the next weeks. I made myself available after hours and checked repeatedly on her progress. Before long she was settled and feeding well, and now at twelve years of age Holly regularly bounds into the practice with her siblings, who also received adjustments.

Holly's case is not rare. As Chiropractors we often encounter people who have been lost in the labyrinth of the current 'sick-care' system or disillusioned by fragmented orthodox care.

The level of care I provided is also not rare. There is such reward in letting clients know we are willing to go the extra mile for them. In our practice we make ourselves accessible to patients by providing our cell phone numbers, particularly to parents who may be prone to anxiety regarding their child's health. It is not uncommon for my husband or me to receive a call from a distressed mother considering taking her child to the Emergency ward, or concerned about a prescription. It is such an honor to be able to talk parents through their fears and have them consider their options. On the rare occasion when the Emergency ward is the best option, parents can still benefit from our support, guidance and care; there are simply times when parents require us to hold their hand.

I believe it is our responsibility as Chiropractors and holistic health practitioners to lead and inspire families towards greater health. We have the skill set, the knowledge, and the resources to do so. If we don't guide families on how to strengthen their health, who will?

Simon and I are blessed to run a health center with a large team of Chiropractors and another ten to fifteen Allied Health practitioners including Chinese medicine practitioners, homeopaths, naturopaths, masseurs, a midwife and lactation consultant, a physiotherapist, and a psychologist, all committed to providing holistic care for families. These wonderful practitioners work together harmoniously, with a patient-centric philosophy, for the common health goal of the client.

Our health center also has a large retail section for stocking organic foods, eco-friendly household products, vitamins, books, etcetera. We desire to create an environment that provides products and services that help guide the health choices of parents. This philosophy has enabled our practice to become a valued resource for families in our community.

Working With Families

Being a parent is tough. Generally speaking we all do the best we can with the knowledge we have at the time, and none of us want to have our choices judged or criticized. Having worked with parents for a number of years now, I have come to realize that like all human beings, parents will go to extraordinary lengths to strengthen their family's health when they feel inspired by extraordinary loving service.

When you work with babies and children, it is my opinion that you need to have a structure in place to allow parents to feel completely supported. It can be very difficult for parents to get an infant to an appointment on time, particularly if they have more than one child, as babies take time to negotiate in and out of cars, dirty diapers happen at the most inopportune times, and toddlers may need additional sleep. Therefore, there needs to be a degree of flexibility in appointment structures. There also needs to be a range of 'family friendly' fee structures, and a comfortable, child-friendly waiting area where parents can relax with other parents and not feel guilty about the noise and chaos that children often make. Toys should be provided, and if possible, additional staff available to take the time to help parents by holding babies, for example. It is also useful to have a quiet breastfeeding area, a change table with nappies and wipes, and child booster seats for the toilets.

Power Of The Adjustment

Sometimes when we are privy to seeing how well the body heals time and time again, we forget to celebrate the miracles we see every day in practice as Chiropractors. Recently an eleven-year-old girl came to see us after suffering with migraines daily for two years. She had gone through every medical test conceivable, and had become so withdrawn her family had even trialed antidepressants. Her history revealed she had suffered a serious knock to her forehead through a sporting accident; our examination and X-ray confirmed this as an AS Occiput subluxation (where the skull is locked down on the upper neck area).

With the first adjustment, this girl's life changed dramatically. When we called her mother later that day, she was so emotionally overwhelmed by the positive changes she could already see in her daughter, she could barely speak. When they returned to the practice two days later, the young girl skipped around the adjusting area in excitement, smiling and engaging in conversation with other clients. Her parents and grandparents, all desperate to understand the power behind the adjustment, accompanied her.

Though we might be tempted to complicate our explanation of adjustments, what Chiropractors do is really so simple: by removing nerve interference and allowing the body to re-calibrate and heal itself, the body is able to express its true capacity for health and vitality. This is much more than just moving joints and bones. Whenever we are practicing, we can strive to maintain our awareness of this power and respect the impact we have on the nervous system.

Health Literacy

Families are unique, and they have unique concerns and needs. It has been my experience that whenever we help parents realize they can navigate their own health outcomes by improving their health literacy, they literally start asking hundreds of health-related questions. Appreciation of health is an invaluable gift to give to parents – and the quality of their health is determined by the quality of questions they ask.

We can encourage conscientious parents to build their health literacy in a number of areas; for example, by looking into what foods may compromise their child's immunity, or by researching the side effects of various drugs. Rather than leaving their health to chance, health literacy determines a family's health culture and the type of health consumer they become.

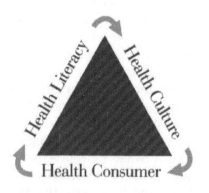

Every Moment Has Infinite Value

Whether we are parents or Chiropractors, health practitioners or support staff, there is no limit to what we can achieve as long as we hold a clear vision. It is up to all of us individually, irrespective of what stage of life we are in, to deeply consider our own health, to create rituals and habits that build self-respect, and to master our thoughts in the present moment.

When we make this commitment to ourselves we begin to see that the influence we can have in our community is unfathomable. We begin to realize we are the path-makers, the catalysts, and the leaders, because happiness and vitality is infectious. By simply opening our hearts to each and every moment, we are presented with ever-replenishing opportunities to be well – in our bodies, in our hearts, and in our minds.

- **Know who you are.**
- **Experience creates wisdom.**
- **Live wholeheartedly.**
- **Live the life you imagine.**
- **We are the company we keep.**
- **Give more than needed.**
- **Every moment has infinite value.**

10

The Universe Provides What I Can Handle
Dr. Andrea Ryan

It is just before nine on a Saturday night and I'm sitting on my couch, trying to put my thoughts to paper as to what I have to contribute to this collection of stories from my colleagues. My two kids are in bed, the youngest is asleep, and our three year old is singing to herself, a song only she understands. This morning, both my husband and I – with our kids in tow – spent a fantastic three hours in the office, serving over twenty-five families during our annual Generation Day. Generation Day is a morning where we celebrate families who choose Chiropractic as part of their lifestyle to keep well. Over seventy-three people were adjusted, one family bringing nine members – grandparents, parents, and children – and to boot, we were missing five members because of other commitments. We then came home and tackled yet another afternoon of home repairs and gardening, doing it on our own – a big undertaking, but a fun learning experience. We topped off the day with a dinner of grilled steaks and vegetables, sitting around a table enjoying the company, stories, and laughs of my family. Looking back, it was a great day. I love these days. A fun balance between my professional life and my family life and I wouldn't have it any other way.

Growing up, from grade eleven forward, I knew two things would come of my future. The first was to go to Chiropractic college and follow in the footsteps of my stepmom, Dr. Liz Anderson-Peacock. The second was to have a family. I had visions of balancing practice and motherhood, with my kids being in the office with me from birth. I could see a family practice bustling with other families coming in for care to keep their loved ones healthy.

Everything Happens For A Reason

Two weeks ago, I was on a plane down to Atlanta, very aware of the deadline to complete my contribution to this book. I couldn't think of what I possibly had to add to such an honourable list of women in Chiropractic. I have been in practice less than eight years and still remember graduation like it was yesterday. The first five years of practice for me were not at all what I expected. They were quite nomadic. I spent a few months in my hometown immediately after graduation and then I practiced in different locations across the tri-state area for about five years. I was learning and growing in my professional life, but I hadn't found what I really wanted or where I really wanted to be. It wasn't until I settled back in Barrie, under a different set of circumstances, that I started to feel settled and attached.

There are two quotes I often reflect back on in my life. The first, "The Universe will only give to me what I can handle." The second, "Everything happens for a reason." Each time I'm faced with something I think is insurmountable I take solace and wisdom from one of these quotes, and very often both of them.

Back to that plane ride to Atlanta: I was headed down south and so excited to see Life University again, for the first time since leaving in 2002, with eight whole years under my belt. Suddenly I realized I *did* have so much to write, so much to share. The balance I want to find between practice and motherhood hasn't yet turned out the way I wanted it to be, but there have been key learning experiences along the way that make me more resolute in what I do as a Chiropractor and a mom.

The first time I took a flight from Toronto to Atlanta, I was a student in grade eleven. I flew down for three days with my stepmom, Dr. Liz, to take in a Dynamic Essentials seminar. I surrounded myself with philosophy, Principled Chiropractors, and was up until two in the morning thinking, "These people are really crazy."

And then I realized I was just as crazy because I was completely moved by Sigafoose talking about a new concept, innate; and I suddenly felt like I had found my purpose in life.

I knew I wanted to be a part of this – part of this force, this excitement that was so infectious it had complete strangers hugging, high-fiving one another, and cheering as each speaker took the stage. Music was pumping through the speakers, my heart was thudding in my chest, and I just knew. I knew this was it. I was going to turn the power on for thousands by something as simple, but yet complex, as an adjustment. I was going to be a doctor of Chiropractic.

I made the decision to go to Life University and started college thinking everyone had to be coming from a very similar up bringing in our profession. Everyone must have had a "Dr. Liz" who introduced him or her to the profession they had chosen. Everyone must be as excited as me to start Chiropractic college, knowing that upon graduation, they would have the most fantastic "job" (if you could call it that) in the world. Everyone would be Principled and on purpose.

Within just a few days of the start of school, my eyes were opened.

I came from small town Canada and here I was in Atlanta. It was exciting meeting people from all over the States, some from Canada (eh!), and even as far away as Mexico, France,

Spain, and South Africa. But just as we all came from different parts of the world, our opinions about Chiropractic were just as varied. I remember sitting beside a guy in my first class and he had never even had a Chiropractic adjustment before. How does one go to college to become a Chiropractor when they hadn't even experienced an adjustment? It just seemed so...*foreign*.

I went through school, enjoying the adventures along the way with new friendships, traveling, jobs, classes, and mentors. I soaked up the philosophy, science, and art of Chiropractic at seminars and started to prepare for being out of school and in practice. Over and over again, I would write down my vision for my ideal practice and draw pictures of the layout I wanted to see. Although, I found the closer I came to graduating, within just a few months, the more anxious I became. Every plan for practice I had planned was solid in my mind, but *where* I wanted to practice was still very cloudy.

Decisions

A large part of my indecision was in light of a new relationship, a young relationship, but a strong one. I met Tom in our first year; we were in the same class together. We didn't start dating until we had six months left in school. He had a fantastic opportunity to go away to Australia for three months and play baseball. So, for over half of our relationship, we were apart. I had the opportunity to go to Australia and visit him for a couple of weeks and when we returned together, our relationship continued to grow. We found common threads in our lives we both loved – staying active through running, biking, swimming, and hiking – yet introduced one another to new experiences, too. If time were on our side, I could see our relationship lasting a while, but with school ending and he from New Jersey and me from Canada, the commitment level was too much for both of us at that point to stick together. When I made the decision to go home, it was by far the hardest one I ever had to make. I had to re-member everything happens for a reason. We filled up my car and drove north, seventeen hours in a car with my cat – to whom Tom had extreme allergies. We spent a week in Canada before saying goodbye in the Toronto airport, for what we both though was for good.

At the time, I thought our relationship was over and I threw myself into practice and into my community. I was back home, practicing with Liz, who was not only my step-mom, but also my professional mentor. As with most new graduates, I had no fear and a hell of a lot of energy. I would say and do anything to build my practice. I participated in health shows, home shows, booths in bookstores, health food stores, and drug stores. I joined a running group and took yoga classes. I became a member of local women's groups, networking groups, referrals groups, and the Chamber of Commerce. I wrote a newsletter. I set up health talks at local groups, organizations, and businesses. I did everything I could to build a practice. I was essentially single, without kids, and could do whatever I needed to do in order to make a success out of my practice. And yes, it grew. Slowly at first, but it seemed like I hit a tipping point where suddenly it took off and referrals were coming in regularly. All of my hard work had paid off and it was so rewarding.

Five months after starting practice, I was on the phone with Tom; we decided being a part was not what either one of us wanted and we started to make plans for our future, both personally and professionally. We missed one another terribly and while the distance between our families was a glaring challenge, ultimately we wanted to overcome it so we could be together. After much deliberation, I made the sec-ond hardest decision of my life – telling the family I loved and respected that we had chosen to make our home together in the States. I was leaving my family and all of the hard work I had done to start another practice.

Thus began our "nomadic" practice experience across Connecticut and New York. Both Tom and I worked with fantastic Chiropractors – Dr. Rick Araya, Dr. Carol Ann Malizia, and Dr. Donna DeRosa – and learned different aspects of practice from each of them. We married in 2005 and decided within a few months to start trying for a baby, as family was important to both of us. We had already talked about children prior to even becoming engaged, so we knew when we did want to have children, we wouldn't have disagreements on the things we both felt were incredibly important to us. We knew we wanted to raise our children in as healthy of a way as possible – sticking to our Chiropractic Principles, trusting that our children would be healthy and that we would support their health with adjustments, good nutrition, and a clean system without the detrimental effects of vaccines or medications.

We went into our pregnancy expecting to have a fantastic, easy pregnancy that would end with a beautiful, healthy homebirth, where we would welcome our child into the world. Little did either of us know the Universe had a very different, very humbling experience waiting for us. For me, this was a time in my life where my Principles and life philosophy were tested. My pregnancy tested my belief system in Chiropractic, and also served as the beginning of setting a stage for a balance between Chiropractic and family.

New Journey – New Lessons

We conceived the first month we tried. It was such an amazing surprise and the start of a great journey. I found out on a Wednesday afternoon, after a positive home pregnancy test (okay, six positive home pregnancy tests). We were thrilled and like any new parents, started to imagine just how amazing it would be to go through pregnancy, and then of course, hold our baby in our arms.

My first trimester went from good to incredibly difficult in a short period of time. About six weeks into pregnancy, I became incredibly ill. It started off slowly: feeling a little dizzy on a treadmill or feeling a bit sick after certain foods. It soon escalated to the point I was throwing up eight to ten times a day, and virtually nauseous any time I was not sleeping. I sat on the bathroom floor and waited for the next time I had to throw up again. The energy required for me to move to my bed or the couch in our living room was just too much. I forced myself to sleep for hours during the day and a minimum of twelve to fourteen hours at night.

The nausea wouldn't subside, and I wasn't able to keep in any food or liquids. Tom typically returned home in the evenings to find me in bed, without enough energy to lift up my head. He literally checked my pulse to make sure it wasn't dangerously low. In just eight weeks, I dropped almost twenty-five pounds and we became really quite nervous as to the health of our baby inside of me. How could it be possible for me to be passing any nutrition whatsoever to a developing baby if I couldn't even keep a multivitamin in my stomach, never mind a meal?

At fourteen weeks, I ended up in the hospital. I had an ultrasound within an hour of being admitted. It was the first of a variety of procedures I didn't initially want nor anticipate in what we expected to be a healthy pregnancy. Although, the ultrasound came with relief when it revealed our baby was developing normally, despite all the challenges I had in the first trimester. I remember a moment of clarity, recognizing that despite the fact neither food nor water had passed my lips without being brought back up for a period of eight weeks, my body managed to continue supporting a baby in growth, and with what appeared to be no problems.

Even though I was extremely dehydrated, our baby was floating in enough amniotic fluid to stay well.

I ended up staying in the hospital for four days, on a continuous IV with anti-nausea medication that helped me regain fluid and healthy weight. Initially, the anti-nausea medication took about eight hours before it kicked-in and I felt the nausea finally subside. A sense of calm spread over me.

My intent to go through pregnancy and labour without medication obviously changed dramatically. I had to let go of the determination of going through it without help, and realize what my body most needed was a break from the stress of hyperemesis (severe morning sickness). And with the relief, everything felt pretty much normal again. I could walk more than ten feet without sitting down to rest. I could drink water without throwing up. I could wake up without getting dizzy and nauseas from rolling over. I was finally able to sit back and enjoy my pregnancy and connect with my baby.

Six months later, early one morning, I woke to the beginnings of contractions. Lying in bed together, Tom and I spent about an hour reveling in the idea that it might be the day we hold our little one. Would it be a boy or a girl? What would the baby look like? *Who* would the baby look like? The anticipation was exciting and it made the initial contractions feel like nothing.

I went from intervals of ten minutes to eight minutes to six minutes in less than three hours. The intensity became incredibly strong and Tom called our midwives and doula, and they arrived shortly after to assist with setting up our apartment to prepare for a healthy, natural homebirth. When my water broke and we saw meconium in the fluid, it was the first indication our baby might have challenges to continue labour as we had planned.

I continued to labour for another few hours after my water broke, but without much progress. The contractions were coming quite regularly, but I wasn't moving along in other areas. I was stuck at 7 cm for over seven hours and regardless of the help from my doula and my midwives, I couldn't seem to get over the plateau. I stayed mostly in my room, feeling calm and in comfort despite the discomfort associated with labour. This was familiar and I could do what I needed to do to deal with the pain. I paced. I went into the fetal position. I was on my hands and knees over a ball. I leaned on my bed. I hung from Tom's shoulders. I could move as I wished, and found the position I had to be in each moment I needed to be there. I could eat and drink as necessary, I sipped on chicken broth and red raspberry leaf infused ice cubes. Each contraction got harder and harder, longer and longer, but at least I was in control of how I dealt with each one. I had to trust my body's innate response to each moment; it was very freeing in that sense.

Honoring The Message By Changing The Plan

I didn't feel like I was in the right place anymore. With such stagnancy at 7 cm for what seemed like so long, I started to get frustrated and even a little scared. I had tried everything I could to get through the last 3 cm – including adjustments – and yet nothing seemed to be working. It was my call, fourteen hours after starting labour with the best intentions of birthing my baby at home without drugs or unnecessary interventions, to transition to the hospital. At best, maybe the hospital setting would calm me enough to allow for me to continue along naturally.

We arrived at the hospital forty minutes later and I was immediately wheeled into a room, put onto an electronic fetal monitoring system, and suddenly the room was filled with a large number of nurses and doctors. From this point on, I don't remember much and I rely on the stories of others to let me know what happened. The obgyn on call came in to do an internal exam, discovering our baby was stressed. The EFM showed the baby's heart was decelerating with each contraction, which meant our baby was under *a lot* of stress and needed to come out as soon as possible.

I do remember thinking a c-section was the last thing on earth I wanted. "This was not in my plan! How did we get here? Why was this happening?"

Looking back, I realize ultimately I lost control of a situation that up until that point – while I let my body do what it needed to do – I had felt in control of, even though it was incredibly painful and exhausting. At that point, in a hospital, the surgeon told me the only option I had was to have this baby through caesarean; I felt very panicked. It took all of ten seconds for the decision to be made, and even before my mom arrived into the room to learn what was happening, I was whisked out and down the hall to be prepped for surgery.

The next hour was a blur. I remember taking a deep breathe and exhaling for the administration of the epidural. I remember lying down, then the sudden loss of sensation of anything below my chest. It was very strange, wanting to move my legs without any success. I remember Tom coming into the surgery room, dressed in scrubs, and holding my hand as it lay strapped to the gurney. I remember crying, thinking I was so far from what I had envisioned, having to put full faith in a surgeon, someone I had never met, as she was about to help bring my baby into the world.

And then, just as in the beginning of my pregnancy, I started to vomit – probably due to the amount of stress my body was under, combined with the drugs required for the surgery. With a mixture of emotions, feeling unprepared, rushed, nervous, scared – and before I knew it, the surgeon announced, "It's a girl!" My heart leaped within my chest.

"A girl! A girl! I had a baby girl." Such excitement, such relief she was out, such fascination to see her. All followed by silence. Silence from this small body that should have made a sound, *a lot* of sounds. No cry. Nothing. She was taken away to a side table and worked upon immediately. Looking back, her APGAR scores were low, very low. She wasn't breathing, wasn't responding, and her heart rate was not good. The nurses and doctors got her to respond within a couple of minutes, but then she was taken from us and put into the Special Care Unit so she could continue to be monitored.

I fell asleep promptly after surgery and was in the recovery room within a few minutes after having her, exhausted from seventeen long hours of labour followed by a heavy dose of meds my body was not used to having. Tom went off to the SCU, and from what I understand it was quite a shock. They had our baby girl hooked up to multiple monitors to check her heart rate, respiration, and blood pressure. She was in an isolet and for a time, Tom couldn't hold her other than to stick his finger in to stroke her leg. We weren't really sure what had gone wrong, or how badly it had affected her. The next forty-eight hours were to tell.

I don't remember much from the recovery room. I remember briefly my mom-in-law being at my side; but I don't remember having a conversation with her. I do remember the surgeon and the nurse discussing me and the surgery and the words along the lines of, "Another half hour and the baby could have died...."

I think I must have drifted back into sleep because the next thing I have any memory of is being in the hallway of the hospital with my family by my side. I was cold and confused, shivering under four layers of blankets, due to the shock of what was going on. I wasn't really aware of the severity of the situation. I think Tom was probably keeping from telling me details until I could register reality a bit better.

My mental clarity was far from clear; all I could focus on was the picture Tom brought to me from the nursery – a picture of a beautiful baby wearing a blue cap. I thought they had the wrong baby, or that they made a mistake when they said it was a girl. Adoringly, Tom went back to the nursery later, asked for a pink cap, and took another picture to prove we did in fact have a girl.

I was taken to the maternity ward and everyone, except for Tom, went home to rest. Tom rested in a cot beside my bed. Two in the morning, we had been up since five the morning before and through an incredibly stressful day. I called my best friend back home to let her know we had our baby, no name yet. When she asked what she looked like, it hit me. I realize that other than a photo of a baby in a blue cap, then a pink cap, I hadn't even had the chance to look at my baby, let alone hold my baby. I suddenly felt so removed and disconnected as her mom.

All the books I had read, the movies I had seen, the stories I heard from other moms painted the picture of joy, as they held their babies moments after coming into the world, bringing their babies to their breast to nurse; I had the image of dad lying beside mom and baby for the first family picture. I didn't have any of that yet. While Tom slept beside me, I stayed awake the entire night wondering what happened and when I would be able to see my little girl. Occasionally, the nurse came in to check my vitals, but other than that it was a long, quiet, dark night with nothing but my thoughts to keep me company. "Is she okay? What went wrong? Why did things end up this way? What did I do wrong?"

Anchoring To Grounding Thoughts For Strength

I started to think back to the two quotes I kept with me for times of distress or frustration. "The Universe will only give to me what I can handle," and "everything in life happens for a reason." With the minutes of the night ticking by, I gathered my composure and started to think about what I was able to do in order to become stronger for myself, as well as what I could do for this little girl. This was an unbelievable test of internal strength. I started to shift from thinking I had done something wrong to cause the situation to instead focusing on what I could do to make things better.

The first thought, my new daughter needed a name. Morning came and I was told I would probably be good enough by about noon to meet our daughter. Tom and I talked, and before family arrived, we decided to name her Caleigh. Caleigh was Gaelic for "celebration," and despite all of the stress surrounding her birth and what we expected we would go through in the next few days, it still was a celebration of life, unity, and family.

I don't think any mom can ever prepare herself for what to expect when going into the special care unit of a hospital to see her child for the first time. Caleigh wasn't premature, but to us she still looked so small and delicate, wrapped up in blankets under heat lamps. She had sensors taped to her arms and a needle in her arm. Sponges were around her hands so that she couldn't pull anything apart or out. By that time, she was stable enough that we could hold her, and so finally, fourteen hours after she was born, I was able to hold my baby in my arms. I will never, ever forget that moment. The first time I looked down at her, into her blue eyes that were so focused and intent on me. We could not take our gaze off one another. It was an instant connection, after so many months of being physically connected; the emotional and spiritual connection for me was now complete. She was there, physically, in my arms and she was perfect.

Two hours later, things once again spiraled downward. Tom and I stood over her isolet and suddenly the horrible sound of alarms started to go off on her monitor. Her breathing was drastically low, so low her tiny hands and feet started to turn blue. The nurses rushed over and immediately started to bring back her respiration to a normal level. What I'm sure was just seconds, no more than half a minute or so, seemed to take forever. They shook her foot, pinched her, and did whatever they could to get her to start breathing. And she did, but what we thought would be just a slow recovery from a difficult birth soon became so much more.

Over the next forty-eight hours, we watched, as she would occasionally stop breathing over and over. Then the mild seizures started, small ones, where her little body would jolt every once in a while. No one could tell us why this was happening. She went on anti-seizure medications, making her body limp as a rag doll. While all new babies have to be supported and cared for, this took it to a new level. Her arms and legs felt so weak, even when held by one of us. The monitors continued to sound off many times and nurses came over to find out what was going on and fix it.

Caleigh went through a battery of tests – EKGs, nerve conduction tests, scans, and more – so many we lost count, and quite frankly, weren't really sure what they were for. No one could identify what was wrong, yet there were plenty of ways to deal with the results of whatever was going on.

Now I was being tested with the biggest test of my life. Certainly, the work of these doctors was vital to Caleigh's survival and I take nothing away from that. I am so grateful for their care. But everything in my training as a Chiropractor taught me to trust in the body's innate ability to heal from the inside out, and to find the *cause* of a problem. I didn't feel the latter was being met, or if it was, it wasn't explained to us. None of the tests performed yielded an answer, yet medications and other procedures were recommended. Treatment with out a diagnosis?

The feeling of letting go and trusting the doctors, accepting they knew what they were doing was difficult. I had to find a way to be involved. So, we took steps that played a vital role in her healing and survival.

Daily, Tom and I adjusted her, making sure her nervous system was functioning as well as possible, to adapt to not only the challenges she was having, but also to recover from the drugs and tests she had to go through. We wanted to make sure our beautiful little girl, born with so much potential had no interference from above, down, inside out. Regardless of what she had to go through to become well, she needed the ability for her body to adapt.

My mom was with me even before going into labour and her love and support for Caleigh and for Tom and I was unparalleled. My other parents – dad, Liz, and my stepdad, George flew down from Toronto to meet their granddaughter and to help out in any way they could, even for moral support. Liz was instrumental in helping me stay focused on my daughter's recovery. She encouraged affirmations, which we did daily. She took the time to adjust Caleigh to make sure her nervous system was free of any interference.

Walking Through Fear

Every meeting with the doctors, every time an alarm went off, every time we encountered a *what if*, I let go of the fear gripping me from inside and instead placed trust in her healing abilities. Everything had to be taken in stride, and it started minute-by-minute, then hour-by-hour, then day-by-day.

The medications were supposed to slowly ware off, within forty-eight hours. On day three, she was taken off the meds, but it took until day nine in the hospital for her to return to normal muscle tone. The doctors needed to see a minimum of twenty-four hours without any monitors sounding. Every time we heard an alarm, our hearts plummeted. We just wanted to make it to that twenty-four hour mark to bring our baby girl home. Ten days later, Caleigh was coming home.

After all of the diagnostic procedures, all of the tests, there was never any conclusive answer as to why she stopped breathing. The seizures were linked back to low blood saline levels. The anti-seizure medication she was on supposedly stopped the seizures; but looking back, coincidentally her seizures stopped around the time she started breastfeeding, too. As an aside, and interestingly enough, her heart is on the right side of her chest and her aorta attaches slightly differently than normal. But that has nothing to do with why she had the challenges she did in the first part of life.

I look back on those ten days in the hospital with our daughter as a huge learning experience. It was humbling. Humbling because what I had planned for my birthing process was far from what actually happened. I realized the best-laid plans with all good intentions could go to the wayside if something is beyond our control. Humbling because where I would love to have a story that a Chiropractic adjustment allowed me to progress through labour successfully, it wasn't a miracle story in this case, this time. But for all I know, those adjustments through labour might have been what kept me well enough to know that it was time to go to the hospital – my innate speaking through me. They could have possibly been what kept Caleigh good enough to be born without further complication. I have to remind myself that everything happens for a reason.

Given The Right Conditions
The Body Knows What To Do

The experience was also awe-inspiring. Awe-inspiring because I watched a seven pound human being, my daughter, fight for her right to live. She had a lot of odds stacked against her and gave us more scares than I could count. Yet each day, she healed and grew stronger. She breastfed on day two perfectly and sucked up as much good nutrition as she could to support her system. She received her adjustments with such ease and her body each time had better communication, better integration. She received love, attention, and positive affirmations from her family both in New Jersey and back home in Barrie, all of which I know made a difference in her recovery.

One would think that such a small person would be frail and unable to cope with the stresses she was under. And yet, she proved that wrong. She wasn't told she couldn't get better or that she couldn't heal. She just did. She had no reason to doubt otherwise. She fought from the moment she was born to get better. Her body knew nothing other than to heal, one step at a time. I have heard stories like this one called miracles, and I assure you that the day we knew we would take her home, in our minds it was. But now looking back, I don't know if it was so much a miracle or just that it just was. It was what it was. I have to remind myself the Universe will only give to me (and her) what we can handle.

Three and a half years later, we now have two beautiful children, Caleigh and Blake. Blake came into this world one year ago today, in fact. We celebrated his birthday this past Sunday with family. He was born by caesarean section too, again due to reasons beyond my control at the time, but before I went into labour. Although, this time around I didn't feel the guilt associated with his birth. I know that everything happens for a reason and the reason behind both my kids coming into the world the way they did makes sense in some way, even though I may never know why.

We also have a beautiful practice, back in Barrie, which we purchased from Liz six months ago. We've bought an amazing family wellness practice and over the next few years, we will bring our own flavour into it, while maintaining its incredible history within our community. For me, finding the balance between home and work actually came fairly easily, although it's constantly being re-assessed. Six weeks after having Blake, I was back in practice with him in tow. He slept at my desk or was held by our CAs or patients while I adjusted people. I managed to fulfill the vision I set forth back in my second year of college. And now on Saturdays, we are sometimes able to enjoy both of us being in practice with our kids, sometimes playing with other kids who come in for their adjustments. Our nanny walks them over to the office on Monday or Wednesday afternoons for their Chiropractic adjustments and they hang around the front office for a while. Caleigh, now three and a half, considers our two CAs as part of her family, often asking where they are and what they are doing when we are at home. My family at home and my family at work are incredibly supportive of one another. If I need to be in my Chiropractic life, I have the support system at home to make that happen. If I need to be Mom, I have an amazing support system at work to allow that to happen. It doesn't get much better than this. While life, practice, and family may not have come the way I initially expected, it happened the way it was intended, and it only makes it that much sweeter now that it is here.

- **I am resourceful.**
- **Anchor to grounding thoughts for strength.**
- **New journeys create new lessons.**
- **Instincts will tell us when to change the plan.**
- **Walk through fear.**
- **Given the right conditions, the body knows what to do.**

11

Living A Life Of Service
Dr. Carol Ann Malizia

You know it is just like breathing... it becomes such a part of who you are and you do it unconsciously. Every now and then you have the beauty and wisdom of a God given moment of truth; you are actually conscious of what you do, like a deliberate long, slow belly breath, the one you took in the first moments of your life and the ones you take when you are finally horizontal after a fourteen hour day.

Truly serving and assisting another's transformation from fear to faith, pain to function without pain, and doubt to hope, for those clients that seek what you do, just like breathing, with effortless ease, is an amazing way to build a life. With the attitude of service, you never work a day in life. Knowing with absolute certainty you can make a difference in people's lives is irreplaceable. Moving any child, man, woman – young, old or infirmed – in the direction of a better quality of life is the greatest reward of a Chiropractors' service, education and mission.

Seeds Of Greatness Are Planted

Healers, true healers have a difference in their spirit, vision and purpose in the world. The seeds of greatness planted in a select few often express themselves, not through their seemingly infinite success or abundant beauty, but to the contrary. It is often through the mud scratching, dig-your-heels-in, guts and courage of the spirit when the seeds decide to grow amidst life's adversities. Life happens when you are busy planning for life, rather than acknowledging the one planned for you by the Universe.

My experience has been that many great healers, teachers and mentors are tested by their own fears, failures and setbacks that mirror the very ones we spend a lifetime helping others move through. There is nothing more painful to a human being than a broken spirit that accompanies a physical or emotional injury.

Likewise, there is little more rewarding than neutralizing, eradicating a pattern in the nervous system created by an injury – either structural or emotional – and replacing a faulty nervous system pattern with a pattern that reflects a vibrant, healthy, happy human being on a path to a better quality of life as a willing participant of your recommendations. We all expose vulnerability when experiencing pain, the affects of a chronic condition, illness or disease. Often a pivotal moment occurs when the doctor knows they can help and communicates that directly with a deep understanding of Chiropractic. The comfort in the confidence, by no surprise, has often been met with tears wept by hundreds of patients who, prior to their time with us, were at the end of their rope, headed for a breakdown – or so they thought.

The power of the connection – a Principle Chiropractic is founded upon – from the very start of my career has been my first love, and a consistent growing love in my entire adult life.

Focus On Others' Needs

Reflecting back, my Chiropractic practice, as in life, has endured many setbacks, though gratefully never any defeats. The unconditional spirit of love and service brought me through many of the hardest days of my human experience.

Because of the great ability to focus on the needs of others, I am able to deter my own temporary pain brought about by life's necessary lessons. I have been taught through Universal Laws that we truly are "spiritual beings having a human experience."

With that in mind, we must come to a realization that our purpose is to assist with clients' movement through the phases of their lives, as well as mirror our own learning from the continuous exchange of energy and experience. The privilege to serve people wherever they are in their world and move them towards a healthier state of being always begins with creating order in their bodies and in their thoughts, ultimately allowing their body to create its own order, even if it involves the order of transition to another form. Our service is certainly not just about relieving symptoms, but rather, to encourage people towards what is destined for them by a higher power. Some of the most amazing moments in practice as a Chiropractor come not with release of pain, but instead with the release of life – delivering an adjustment to allow the body the ease to take its next breath again, a breath of a better life.

Studying the patterns of my clients over a twenty-one year period has fascinated me. Clients become their patterns of structure, nutritional habits and thought. Combined, that leads to a culmination of events that may appear as a painful interruption and annoyance to their habits and responsibilities of daily living. Training the body through regular Chiropractic adjustments, supported by whole food nutrition and healthy thinking, has created some of the most profound transformation in healing and restoration of function I have ever witnessed.

The body, in its wisdom has never let me down; it always knows what it is doing, even if the client gets sick after an adjustment: it is the bodies innate wisdom telling the body to rid itself of the toxic overload that potentially has created the issue in the first place. Understanding it is not always pleasant for the patient, to say they went home and tossed their cookies, or had the bowel movement that rivaled passing a Rattan wicker chair after an adjustment. However we now embrace the understanding that a Chiropractic adjustment facilitates the balance in the organism, in ANY SHAPE or FORM to restore the physical body's ability to adapt. This premise is the basis for ill-health; when the organism can no longer adapt to its environment from physical, chemical and emotional stressors that break the system down. In its wisdom, the body knows how to correct itself when given the opportunity for better function by relieving the stressors placed on the system.

Vision: An Influential Tool

A key to facilitating hope and positive change in others is to share with them a vision in their future that is greater than the one they currently hold of themselves. The vision we have for ourselves and for others is one of the most powerful tools we were ever granted in our human experience. It is free of charge and can bring us to any state of physiology, emotional shift, or conscious agreement with ourselves at any given moment we decide to participate.

I have recollections of practicing in my earlier years, in a high volume atmosphere, just focusing on the vision of a beam of light that permeated out of every skull. This light lit up the spinal cord as I palpated down every spine. Interruptions of light were so obvious when I was looking for them, looking without my eyes.

Intuition, gut feelings, and nudges from above – or from wherever your belief system believes those split second 'knowings' originate – are the most powerful voice among the chatter. The trick is to develop enough self-esteem and confidence to trust that voice and dismiss any arising doubt from knowing. The vision of what is happening inside a body under your hands is a form of this very 'knowing.'

Quieting the mind to focus on this vision, without the conscious mind jumping in to chatter, is paramount to the success of the visualization process. Chattering of the mind is where we discovery our enemies of doubt, worry and fear. This is why the concept of clinical excellence, certainty and present time consciousness (PTC) are necessary ingredients to combine with vision.

Gain Clarity Through A State Of Inner Calm

Question and doubt breed unhappiness from the uncertainty and worry they create. In my experience, I have come to realize my speed through life was quite often motivated by fear and doubt. When I learned to slow down, clarity was the by-product of a state of calmness. Breathing and healing generally facilitate one another. Building trust and confidence that there is a greater plan at work, even though you may be faced with an extraordinary amount of chaos, is all part of the grand organizing design for our evolution. The plan does not always come in a time frame we are comfortable with, nor through a circumstance we see at the time as necessary. However, it will provide time for reflection, responsibility and gratitude.

These events may provoke great change, and pain along our journey. They trigger the proverbial 'pebble in the pond' cascade of events and changes we are not always ready to face.

There was an experience early in my career that stopped me in my tracks, and later reminded me of the power of this 'pebble in the pond.' It was about four in the afternoon and the office was in motion, I mean cranking: moving in and out of rooms, assisted by a staff that functioned like a well oiled machine, attending to all our clients needs to insure their visit to our office was the best part of their day.

In I went to room two. As I flew in, processing information in my mind from the previous patient, I am greeted by familiar faces: Anne – the mother and dedicated Chiropractic referral machine, her son Jason – an outstanding athlete with a full punch-card for trips to the local Emergency room prior to finding Chiropractic, daughter Jessica – an equally talented athlete with the compromise of a scoliosis. Almost immediately my perception changed, felt through my skin. Something was not right. Before my mind could catch up to my goose bumps and the perception that something was not right, Anne remarked, "Dr. Carol, please adjust the kids first, me last, and then I need you to sit down for a minute." Jessica was already on the table.

The pit in my stomach appeared immediately and felt queasy, confirming the goose bumps. I did as Anne requested, and then sat down.

Anne looked in my eyes and expressed how grateful she was for being able to bring the kids here for a Chiropractic adjustment to relieve their immediate stress, and prayed in the future it would some how offset the tragedy they were about to face. Mike, Anne's husband and the kid's dad, was just pulled out of Hudson River, dead, and the coroner contacted them to identify the body.

Where do I go from here?

The reception room is full of eager clients, patiently waiting.

In front of me, a family with such a sobering reality filled with overwhelming grief, and yet their enormous belief structure that their mental and physical bodies were so much more capable of handling their level of stress with an adjustment prior to identifying their Dads' body, they came to be adjusted first.

In that moment I was so humbled to the burdens of this family and prayed there was more I could do to offer support. This family has been a precious part of my practice for twenty-one years, however the greatest gift came years later.

Much of my free time I select to spend teaching others about the purpose of service within a Chiropractic practice. On such a day, I was teaching to a large group of Chiropractic Assistants in Atlanta, Georgia. At the end of my presentation there was much chatting in the front of the room, and I noticed a large, young handsome figure fill the frame of the door in the back of the room. As he came closer to me, I could not help but keep looking, there was an energy so familiar, yet so out of place. Out of his mouth came, "Dr. Carol Ann, its me Jason! I heard you were in our neck of the woods down here, and I thought I would drop in and tell you what a great life I have, because I became a Chiropractor! I practice right here in downtown Atlanta, and I just wanted you to know what an influence you have been on my life!"

POW!!! Now that was what I call an 'Ahhh-ha moment.' What a lump in my throat to know this talented young gentleman went on to practice what I practice, and dedicate himself to a life of serving humanity in a way that will now change others' lives as I have had the privilege.

So, you see, living a life of service driven by a purpose is a road filled with the abundance of opportunities to move struggling human beings through a place in their life, and allows the doctor of connection/Chiropractic to transform the stress of life into the breathe of life. It creates the ability to say "YES" to change, to say "YES" to circumstances that would seem insurmountable, and allows all to see the other side of those circumstances as blessings within those circumstances, often delivering the ultimate healing at the right moment we are awakened.

If stress were not consistently being removed from our bodies and minds, we would miss some of the most invaluable experiences that shape our future and who we are in that future. Being blessed with the gift to assist people in their experience of being human is second to none, and comes with the responsibility. Influencing hundreds and hundreds of lives over the years, and instilling the one ingredient we all need more of in life: hope.

The side benefit of a lifetime of helping others is the great chance to get to know yourself. Some of our deepest struggles almost appear laughable once the years and sting of the pain have past. I believe we create in our life some of the darkest times, to not only learn about ourselves, but in turn to develop a deeper understanding for others when they experience ups, downs and temporary derailments in their life.

Emotional upheavals prove to me over and over again, that in the end we always have the choice over what has dominion over us; truly the only power anything or anyone has over us is the power we give it. The energy of our beliefs, more importantly the energy of our negative beliefs, can keep us stuck in cycles of sameness until we choose between the pain of the same, or the pain of change. Thus, defining moments of my life have not always been when the sun was shining, looking in the mirror at a perfect size four suit, plenty of money in the bank, the love and unconditional devotion of spouse and family. This chic-gene is a tricky one.

As a leader of a practice, balancing the business energy with the energy of a male/female relationship creates an interesting platform for learning. I, for one, experienced both extremes; from dressing like a man – suits/ties/briefcases, cutting my hair very short, doing what my perception told me was necessary, to stepping out of my comfort zone, into a circumstance of sheer femininity to the opposite extreme.

Well, how was that working for me?

Needless to say, that manifested a boat load of insecurities leading me to a greater desire for my inside to match and be congruent with the outside, no matter what the circumstances were on the outside, including my weight.

I Am Fully Equipped

After many years of studying the Laws of Attraction, and focusing on women from other cultures, I became fascinated with why so many of my colleagues suppressed their femininity in exchange for professional/corporate upward mobile positioning. It spurred me to seek female role models from other walks of life, professions, disciplines and cultures. Amazingly after many, many years of the 'not-enough syndrome,' I found myself studying women whose attitudes and beliefs were that they came fully equipped.

I began to embrace the fundamental principle that my femininity is an attribute, and without a doubt, my soul did not have a gender or size, only a purpose. Although, as time rolls by I am delighted I am a part of the gender with the shoes and purses! Ironically, I have come to appreciate the simplicity of life, the choices and the attitudes, with gratitude.

I have come to understand anything we focus our mind on with enough emotion will manifest. Even the bad things in life, if reinforced over and over with thought patterns, will be etched into the nervous system. This is why the power of freeing the nervous system of its interferences' has become such a critical choice in health care. Removing interference provides our mind with the ability to make better choices to process pain, disappointment and anger. When we participate in regular Chiropractic care, as I have witnessed in nearly tens of thousands of cases, we can manage rather than be owned by our feelings and thoughts. The transfer of energy in and around the body through the mind is the most essential component to all healing.

I love to live by the adage that the best of you is ahead of you, and teach clients that the body and mind always have an opportunity for repair and rejuvenation, no matter the circumstances. Just like breathing, we do it unconsciously; and just like helping others, it truly is the breath of life for a life with purpose.

- **Seeds of greatness are planted.**
- **Focus on others' needs.**
- **Vision is an influential tool.**
- **Gain clarity through a state of inner calm.**
- **We are fully equipped.**

The Time Is Now
Dr. Claudia Anrig

One of my biggest life lessons from my parents was, I could achieve whatever I put my mind to – there were no limits for the goals I could set for my life. They did say it would take work, but as a child I was given the chance to think big and was brought up with no limitations. I guess because of that up bringing I never saw a glass ceiling, just an opportunity for a *first.*

I was introduced to Chiropractic care when I was very young. My mom is one of those Chiropractic miracle stories we often hear. When she was pregnant with my younger sister, Susi, she began to suffer with debilitating lower back pain and went the medical route. Doctors told her once she gave birth, the pain would ease up; but she gave birth and the pain just got worse. The medical profession basically told her to learn how to crawl and bear weight as little as possible.

My mom's situation went on for months, with my dad working all day and also acting as Mr. Mom at home. While my dad was at the store one day, the gentleman at the counter inquired about his wife and kids, mentioning he hadn't seen them in a while. My dad, normally a very quiet man, shared what was happening to my mom, and the man said immediately, "She has to go see a Chiropractor."

Back then, my parents – immigrants from Switzerland – couldn't even pronounce the word, let alone spell it. Yet, they were looking for hope, so they went to the Chiropractor the next day. He examined, x-rayed, and began adjusting my mom. Within a few weeks, she was out of pain. Just a few short weeks later, she could walk again; and so, as often happens, she stopped going.

My parents, tired of shoveling snow, decided to move to Arizona. About a year and a half later, my mom's pain returned. As all Chiropractors know, most people don't understand you have to stay with adjustments even when there's no pain.

My mother's condition deteriorated horribly; so, since the first one helped so much, she decided to go back to a Chiropractor. Again, she was examined, x-rayed, and adjusted, and within just a few weeks she was pain free, walking again. But the difference between the two experiences was education.

The Power Of Communicating The Story

The Chiropractor took the time to tell my mom she had between phase-two and phase-three spinal degeneration; and for her spine to be like this in her early 30's the problem had to have begun when she was a child. She also remembered having back pain and leg cramps as a young girl. These later developed into severe menstrual cramping; and thanks to the Chiropractor's explanations and his health care class, my parents realized that because my mom's problem began in childhood, they should bring their children in for care.

I was between the ages of five and six when I received my first Chiropractic adjustment. A year or so later, when my parents asked me what I wanted for my seventh birthday, I told them I wanted a set of full spine x-rays so I could take them to school and teach my classmates why all children need Chiropractic care. Dr. Guest, my Chiropractor at that time, thought that was such a fabulous wish he gave me those x-rays as a birthday gift. I took them to school and gave my class a three-day lay lecture on the benefits of Chiropractic care. At this young age I knew I was going to be a Chiropractor.

My dad, an engineer at the time, was also very moved by our experience with Chiropractic. He decided to change careers and we moved to Los Angeles, where he enrolled in Cleveland Chiropractic College. Once in a while, a Friday 'family night' with my dad consisted of going to classes with him. It was a wonderful time, and as a kid I loved Chiropractic. I loved going to the seminars with my parents; the whole family would sit in the front row with a pad and pen and take notes. I guess it's no surprise my brother, Daniel, and my sister, Susi, are Chiropractors now as well. We have a family practice all together and my mom is our office manager.

Not seeing a glass ceiling didn't start with my career. My mother is an excellent example of someone who would not let glass ceilings limit her or her potential. Over sixty years ago, when it was unheard of for a woman to be in any position of responsibility or authority, my mother was a manager at a retail establishment – a definite first. Initially she wasn't receiving equal pay for her work. But after a year, she spoke to the president of this multi-million dollar company and let him know she intended to quit if she was not compensated for her value; she received the salary increase she was due – another first.

I think this explains why, when I started Chiropractic college and was told the technique I wanted to pursue was too difficult for women, I didn't let it stand in my way. My upbringing taught me I could achieve whatever I wanted, as long as I was willing to work hard enough to accomplish it. I couldn't fathom how a few inches of plumbing could hinder someone from learning a technique, so I applied myself and became a master Gonstead Chiropractor.

During that era, there were few, if any women in attendance at seminars. It wasn't unusual for me to be the only woman, but I wanted to develop my skills and give back to the technique that helped my mother walk again. So I did what I had been raised to do: I didn't take "no" for an answer. I worked hard to achieve my dreams. I became the youngest and first American woman to become a Diplomat and Fellow of the Gonstead Clinical Studies Society – a level of technical and clinical proficiency tested by peers.

Filling A Void

As a teenager attending seminars with my father, and also as a Chiropractic student, I was always keenly aware of the lack of women on the major platforms. In the late Eighty's, I was traveling with my dear friend and colleague, Judy Forrester from Calgary. We discussed the obvious void. We decided then and there it was time to see women teaching, so we planned to host our own seminar. A year later we taught the first twelve-hour comprehensive family seminar called, Peter Pan Potential, which we taught well into the mid-Nineties.

We taught thousands of doctors and their staffs the science, education and philosophy of a family practice. This was an amazing time of awareness for our colleagues. Even today, I have doctors come to me and share that they became a Chiropractor or decided to turn their focus to family care because of the 'intention' Judy and I brought to our profession.

Even today, the educational products from Peter Pan Potential continue to serve our profession worldwide. When an educational tool is directed from a woman to reach out to women and their families, the results are slightly different. All I can say is that is works.

As the first woman board member for the Gonstead Clinical Studies Society – a non-profit organization dedicated to promoting teaching and research – I became the first woman president. With hard work and dedication, I knew I could affect change with my desire to move the profession forward. In this role I began to really influence the technique I loved so much. We were growing as an organization, delving deeper into research, and in the midst of all this I was published in a Chiropractic textbook edited by Dr. Gregory Plaugher.

I feel an awesome sense of appreciation when I see the technique is now being used by thousands of women; and many of them are advancing the work: Phyllis Markham, Jeannie Taylor, Linda Mullin, Susi Anrig, Susan Caruso, Monika Buerger, Muriel Perillat, Cherie Goble, and Lydia Dever, just to name a few.

It was also a distinct honor of mine to bring the Gonstead Technique officially to Australia in 1990. With nine doctors donating their time and expenses to teach in Sydney, my friend and colleague, Dr. Peter Walters and I arrived to a sold-out seminar and launched the Australian Gonstead Chiropractic Society.

Say Yes When Opportunity Arises

One of the most deeply gratifying experiences in my life has been my relationship with my dear friend, Larry Webster, the founder of the International Chiropractic Pediatric Association (ICPA). I was the first one he asked to be a board member, and our first collaboration was the creation of the certification program, now evolved into one of the largest ongoing certification programs worldwide. Probably one of the most important but rewarding decisions I made years ago was not accepting Larry's invitation to take over the association. At the time, my gut told me this was bigger than one or two people and I encouraged him to expand the board

– and he did. It was a huge transition, but I was honored, with the passing of our dear colleague, to be able to say I was the first woman president of the ICPA.

The ICPA is an amazing non-profit organization and, as a whole, brings with it many firsts. It is the largest family Chiropractic based association, lead by an amazing executive director, Jeanne Ohm. It is the first pediatric based association to have a full time researcher, Joel Alcantara, and it currently provides the largest Chiropractic public outreach with the magazine *Pathways* and the informational public website, www.icpa4kids.org.

I personally believe this organization is leading our profession into a future where parents don't hesitate to take their children to a Chiropractor and women recognize immediately the benefits of prenatal Chiropractic care.

In 1994, I was first contacted by Lippincott, Williams and Wilkins regarding editing a pediatric textbook. It was a pretty amazing invitation and I accepted without hesitation but with one stipulation: I wanted to co-edit with Dr. Gregory Plaugher. And so, with blood, sweat and a lot of tears, the *Pediatric Chiropractic* textbook was released in 1997 and has been the fastest selling textbook in our profession. This book has been used worldwide in Chiropractic colleges and in a clinical setting by practicing doctors. With the second edition being released in 2010, we expanded the textbook by 30 percent and our fellow women co-authors from four to eleven.

Shortly after the textbook was initially published, I began to receive numerous requests by young doctors asking me if they could shadow me in my practice. They always had the same question, "How do you grow and maintain a successful family practice and how can I do that, too?" Since I continue to run a full time, high volume practice, it was difficult for me to think about the logistics, but I was moved by the requests and a desire to help out with the needs of my colleagues.

This was the birth of a mentoring program designed by a woman to teach doctors how to educate their patients and move their practice from relief-based to wellness-focused. What is unique about this two-year program is I only mentor forty doctors a year and it is intimate – there are no other coaches. I keep it very real and never suggest to anyone to do something I am not currently doing in my own practice.

What has made *Generations* work for my doctors world-wide is our focus on education and lifestyle information for parents wanting to raise healthy families. Utilizing educational tools and protocols that I've used successfully in my own practice, I have helped doctors – whether new to the profession or practicing for twenty years – educate their patients as to the benefits of Chiropractic care for whole families.

As a mentor, I've had the unique experience of watching a doctor who was afraid to express the importance of the care she was offering, suddenly become strong and secure in her identity as a Chiropractor. I have another wonderful woman who has been with my program for over four years, who *swore* when she began with me that she would never lecture in her community. Since then, she's become a popular guest speaker and now advocates to fellow Chiropractors the importance of getting the message out into your community with speaking engagements. It's changed her whole outlook on the effect you can have through education.

However, I believe that one of the most important things we, as women Chiropractors, can do for our colleagues is offer support to those who are having children. In developing personal relationships with the doctors in my *Generations* program, I've witnessed the struggle to balance having a child and maintaining a practice at the same time. It's not unusual to hear women talk about the difficulty in balancing family and career; but as a Chiropractor, that balance can be even more challenging since their goal is to raise a wellness family. This may require sacrificing time from their practice to achieve their personal goals for their family and will sometimes elicit feelings of misplaced guilt. As not just a mentor but also a friend, I am along for the journey with them.

My deepest satisfaction comes from seeing doctors have their 'moment of awareness' – that moment when they realize their dreams and recognize they can have the family practice they've always wanted. I believe the doctors in my program already have what it takes, but it may require a different kind of mentoring relationship to bring it out.

Probably the biggest compliment I could've received came in 2006, when my first *Generations* class was ready to graduate. They informed me they weren't ready to stop and asked if I would continue to teach them. It took some time, but I started *Next Generations* for the graduates, and I'm blessed that these colleagues remain a part of my life.

Influence Of Mentors

The amazing thing about the word 'mentor' is that it can be a person or an action. There have been people in my life who have influenced my goals and the decisions I've made simply by being who they are and how they live. There are still others who have actively mentored me and made themselves a part of my life.

There is an amazing energy produced when you choose to align yourself with people who have the same goals and dreams that you do – and it can spill over into every aspect of our profession. It's a matter of joining our hearts and creating an alliance based on what we want to bring to the future of Chiropractic. This can be our legacy – education and information without the drama.

Sure, it may seem like I'm saying that we can have it all, but what's wrong with that? With the right balance in our lives and the right people on our side – it's not impossible. Understanding that as professional women and doctors you are expected to make it all work and be successful; it's a matter of finding your focus, aligning your priorities with your dreams, and taking it all one step at a time.

I believe the future of Chiropractic will pivot to appeal more and more to families when more women realize they have so much to offer our profession on a local, state, national and international level. Look at your strengths and see how you might use those skills and resources to grow our profession, and yet maintain our inherent roots. To move away from the Principles of Chiropractic – that we are a science, art and philosophy – is to invite the erosion of our foundation, leaving us with nothing.

Whether you are a Chiropractic student, a Chiropractic mom balancing life or a veteran, we can all give at one level or another to the profession. My mother has always said, "The profession has given us much and we need to give back to the profession." This statement is more true now than ever before – to see our profession continue to grow it will need nurturing. This effort will take the will of many... and I would suggest the will of many women.

How can we give back to our profession? If you are a Chiropractic student, donate time to clubs on your campus or promote your college by volunteering to speak to potential students. More than anything, just having a spirit of gratefulness for all the instructors and administrators that diligently serve to provide you the tools you need to graduate, will promote Chiropractic. None of us will have the perfect college experience, but a kind word or a thank-you note will go further than you know.

If you are a young Chiropractor without a lot of funds, you can give back by volunteering on a local or state level for your association. You could be a guest speaker for a campus club or host a Chiropractic student(s) at your practice or home so they can afford to attend a seminar.

When we have been blessed with practice growth, often we have the financial means, but not the time. In this case, you can support our profession in a variety of ways: contact your college alumni association and offer to sponsor the tuition of a student, or help a young doctor to attend a conference or pay for their first year membership. Your options are really limitless. Perhaps you're especially blessed and you have a successful practice and still some time; if this is the case and you are gifted in the area of strategic thinking or can see ways an organization could move forward, you may have a calling for politics in our profession. Consider a board position at a Chiropractic college or non-profit organization, especially one related to research in your technique.

If you feel comfortable instructing or have a desire to lecture, you may find yourself back at a Chiropractic college or teaching your own seminar someday. If you're a gifted writer, this may be an opportunity to publish articles or even your own book. It could be that your dream is to see the science in our profession or your particular technique grow; if so, contribute to publishing research.

Many times we think we don't have the time or resources to give back, but this is rarely the case. We can always find ways to give back to a profession that has given us so much. Look for those opportunities, even in the smallest way, keep an eye out for every chance to advance. Each ounce of energy and intention we give to the profession can be the catalyst to shift not only our profession, but also those lives that come into contact with us.

- **There are no limits to your goals.**
- **Achieving goals takes discipline and hard work.**
- **Communicate the story.**
- **Say yes when opportunity presents itself.**

Manifest Your Destiny
Dr. Grace Syn

I thought I was on route to fulfill my dreams to be a trial attorney. Sitting in my undergrad class (Italian 101) at California State University Long Beach, my classmate asked a question that changed the course of my life: "My boss needs a back office assistant, do you want a job?" I asked what kind of office it was, and she replied Chiropractic.

I was always into health and fitness, but at that time I hadn't a clue what Chiropractic was or did. I went down to hang out with the doctor and was blown out of the water with what I saw. People were coming in sick and leaving better. Grandmas were walking in bent forward and walking out upright. Dockworkers with debilitating pain left with a smile. Babies with colic were adjusted and stopped crying. The quality of life improvement through Chiropractic was nothing short of amazing to me. I applied for the job and worked in that office for two years mainly because I really wanted to be in that environment. At that time, I changed my major from Political Science to Health Science and decided to pursue Chiropractic.

Well, the time had come to visit both of the southern California Chiropractic colleges. Cleveland Chiropractic College was a four story building in lovely smog ridden Los Angeles. They had a great cafeteria though, with awesome food. LACC (now SCUHS) in Whittier had a campus with grass, a track, a gym, a lot of *all* hot guys, but no cafeteria. They only had a lunch truck – good ol' Bocho's meals on wheels. What is a girl to do? Of course I went where all the hot guys were. I got a good academic education at LACC, but it wasn't necessarily a Chiropractic education. Philosophy was not a strong point.

Defining Moments Of Truth

I graduated in December of 1992 and didn't have the *darndest* clue about what I wanted, where I wanted to go, and how I was going to grow my practice. Luckily, I had two doctors fighting over me to be their *paid* extern while I waited to become licensed. Somehow I found myself in the middle of a bidding war; the highest bidder won and I ended up back in my old neighborhood where I grew up, Redondo Beach.

I'm not going to sugar coat it, when I arrived at my new office, it was not such a great experience. I soon found out the real reason why I was hired. I was asked by my boss to wear short skirts and attend work comp attorney's luncheons to get more business. Then I witnessed our office manager in tears because he was screamed at to bill whatever he can find (even though some were not legitimate charges) to get her another ten thousand dollars to buy a boat. As a rookie, my heart was broken. This was not what I thought I was signing up for.

I called my father in crying, not knowing what I should do. 'Bank of Daddy' to the rescue. He told me to get out of that toxic place and find a new office. In the meanwhile, 'Bank of Daddy' took good care of me. And so I did, I found a new office on the other side of town. This time, I made an agreement to work on a 60-40 (owner/me) percentage, instead of salary, and continued my externship. I was a bit green in business negotiation skills and had no clue that I was not making a good deal for myself. Being a young, small statured, female doctor, it was a challenge for people to take me seriously. I was asked by one of the other doctor's patients if I was the interior decorator for the office. I guess he saw me moving my furniture in and just assumed.

Moving From Frustration To Motivation

I sat in my office slower than molasses and thought, "When are all my new patients going to walk through the door? Don't they know that I'm here?" And so I sat many days bored and not busy. This gave me plenty of time to study for the Boards. At that time, California state boards were all oral. Four days of pure anxiety. Thank God I passed the first time through! After boards I was a bit rounder than I was used to being because all I did was eat and study for six straight months. I definitely did not fit into my *skinny* jeans by any means and I certainly wasn't impressed with myself naked. It was time to do something about it. So I acquired a new hobby and picked a new goal. I decided I was going to do a *Miss Fitness USA* competition. I hired a gymnastics coach and a trainer to kick my buns into tip-top condition, dialed in my nutrition, worked-out two times a day and was in fabulous shape.

After receiving my license, I decided it was time to move on and I found an office that had four Chiropractors, one orthopedist, one neurologist, and a plastic surgeon. This time it was a 50-50-percentage agreement. I learned how to manage PI, Work Comp, and Insurance cases. After three years of this type of practice, I felt my skills as a Chiropractor was just okay, but not extraordinary. I found myself frustrated, burned out and still struggling to make ends meet. I was miserable. I was seriously contemplating leaving the profession at this point.

When The Student Is Ready, The Teacher Will Appear

During this time, I met a Principled Chiropractor at my gym, Dr. Tim Stakis, who invited me to his Health Talk at his office. I went, not knowing what to expect. He rocked my world when he said: "Subluxations kill!" I realized I didn't fully understand subluxations or the devastating effects of them up until that point. At that time, I didn't have the certainty or courage to say that to any of my patients, but I knew in my heart I had to be different from that point forward.

I gave notice at the office. Not knowing where I was going, I knew I was definitely leaving but was going to stay in the area. There's a part of my town called the Riviera Village that is absolutely beautiful. It's where the beaches meet the hills. This area had boutiques, restaurants, surrounded by palm trees and is right next to the beach. I saw this gorgeous four-story corner business building with underground parking. I said to myself, *"Someday."* I learned at that time if you make a decision on having something and put it out there, it will come.

I was working out at the gym and a lady came up to me and introduced herself. She was an acupuncturist and heard I may be looking for space. I said I was, and she said, "I own a building in the Riviera Village and have a really cute 500 sq. ft. office that you may like."

I went by to see it and fell in love with it. It was teeny-tiny, but it would be all mine. The lobby had just enough room for two wicker chairs, the bathroom was inside the adjusting room and everyone had to 'hold it' until the person inside was finished with being adjusted. I had half a front counter and a fax/phone machine to conserve space. I didn't have much money and started my new solo practice on a credit card.

So off I went, I started my new practice with me, myself, and I. All three of us were ready to work hard. It was sink or swim for me. For the first six months I busted my buns telling everyone I knew in the area that I opened up shop and to come to have their spine checked. Then I made enough money to hire someone part time. I became busier and gave her full time work. I grew that little practice in two years and

I was at max capacity for that little space. It was time for me to move.

I got into my car, turned the corner and saw a great 890 sq. ft. office space for lease. It was perfect for what I needed. I called the owner and scheduled an appointment to see the place. A little, four-foot eight-inch old lady with blue hair came walking up. We introduced ourselves and I saw the available space. She asked what I did, and I told her I was a Chiropractor. Her face soon changed expression and she told me her last tenant was a Chiropractor and she hated him. He ruined the suite by spilling x-ray processing solution all over the place and not cleaning it up properly. I said to her, "Mrs. D, I can't speak for the last doctor but I can tell you what I'm about. My purpose is to help as many people resolve their health issues and get healthy without the use of drugs or surgeries. There are too many sick people out there getting sicker due to the side effects of medications."

She looked at me and said, "Here are the keys; I like you." I was stunned. No credit check, no application, she just handed me the keys. She said, "I'll draw up a contract and you can sign it later. In the meanwhile you can start your build out."

I was so excited!

Pivotal Moments

#1. I realized I needed help in growing my practice to the next level. I was looking through a Chiropractic trade publication and saw an advertisement for The Prescott Group (now known as The Chiropractic Business Academy). The ad listed names of some of their clients and how well they were doing. One of the names I recognized. Normally I would've been skeptical, but it happened to be a person I knew and had dated. I called him and he said it was true. He said he did collect that much in a month. I was more than impressed and called the company to find out more. I spoke to Dr. Lori Prescott. She was a woman who could teach me a thing or two, since she already had accomplished what I wanted. She was a mother, a wife, and had a million dollar practice. I signed on as a client and tripled my gross in three months. I learned the difference between corrective Chiropractic care and pain management. I then saw the need to learn more. I sought out posture correcting techniques like Pettibon and CBP. The key was being able to produce results and quantify outcome measurements. I learned how to educate my patients properly so they saw the value in being under care. I finally had systems in place and learned how to grow my business *deliberately.*

Since then, my practice has grown exponentially. Remember the '*someday*' building? I grew my practice big enough to be able to move into a 2,700 sq. ft suite in that '*someday*' building and serve even that many more people. I've just expanded that office to a beautiful 4,400 sq. ft integrative family wellness center that teaches people how to "Be Fit, Eat right, and Think Well." I used to call Dr. Bill Demoss's office the "Taj Mahal" of Chiropractic because it is so beautiful. I now call my newly expanded center "Taj Mahal 2.0."

#2. I put into the Universe that I wanted to see more kids (but just didn't know how). I knew I wanted to have more specialized training in pediatric Chiropractic. I saw an advertisement for a Chiropractic pediatric summit in Washington DC, so I went. That weekend changed the course of my practice. I met Dr. Patrick Gentempo, who is now one of my most invaluable and cherished mentors. I saw this incredible computerized analysis to measure subluxations. I thought, "Wow!" I was scanned and saw how *jacked-up* my system was. I was asked if I would like to purchase it and I said yes. The next thing I knew, I was filling out paperwork, *bada-bing-bada-boom*: a proud owner of an Insight Millennium Subluxation Station™.

Generally speaking, I usually make pivotal decisions in a New York minute and don't vacillate. Patrick said, "See you at the mountain." Little did I know the impact going to "the mountain" was going to have on my practice. "The mountain" is a Chiropractic boot camp/sub-station training in the Colorado Mountains called "Total Solutions." This is a *must* for any DC. It turned my world inside out, upside-down in a great way. The Chiropractic message was *roto-rootered* through me beyond measure. By far, it was *the* most pivotal Chiropractic experience for me...ever. I came off the mountain like Moses with white hair and the ten commandment plates. I saw the light and was never the same again. I *got* Chiropractic and my purpose was set on fire like a burning inferno.

#3. At the mountain, I met Dr. Steve Hoffman. What a cool dude. He taught me a technique that has forever changed the lives of every patient that walks through my doors. When I learned the MC2 (Mastering Chiropractic with Certainty) technique, it changed whom I attracted into my office. Complicated cases like birth trauma babies and seniors were showing up at my door step. No one ever told me that there was something called a Tonal technique. All I knew was the manual stuff. The manual techniques are great, but there is a time and a place. I am now a certified MC2 instructor and teach this wonderful technique to others.

#4. A few years ago, I became curious about cranial adjusting. It's not something taught in our schools nor do many of us practice with it. I started to think, if the CNS is made up of the brain and spinal cord, how come we only adjust the spine? Well, the Universe heard my question loud and clear and sent me some educational material in the mail about training for cranial adjusting. It was called C.A.T.S. (Cranial Adjusting Turner Style). Dr. Rodger Turner is a Canadian Chiropractor who taught me how to adjust the cranium. All I can say is "Oh my God." It is one of the most powerful tools in my tool bag as a Chiropractor.

Baby Evan

I was referred an eighteen month old boy named Evan. Evan was a c-section/forceps baby. He couldn't hold his own head up and was born crossed eyed. His ophthalmological surgeon was recommending Evan go under surgery to cut cranial nerve III to 'correct' his crossed eyes. I told his parents I cannot guarantee anything; however based on my exam findings their child was severely subluxated. I asked if it was possible for them to hold off on the surgery for one month and see what we can do Chiropractically. They agreed to go the Chiropractic route.

During Evan's fourth week of care, his mom came into the office first while dad was parking the car. She was crying. I asked what was wrong and she said it was tears of joy. She said Evan was able to focus on his *Baby Einstein* video for forty-five minutes. As dad and Evan walked into the office, I noticed Evan wasn't crossed eyed anymore. We all cried together. Needless to say, Evan did not undergo any surgery.

Geraldine

An eighty-four year old 'hot tamale' named Geraldine came in for a consultation. She said, "I really don't have any issues but some neck stiffness" (though her medication list indicated otherwise) "and came in upon the insistence of my granddaughter." Her granddaughter was already a client of mine.

Geraldine saw her scan and x-ray findings, saw a 42 degree curvature in her thoracic spine, and asked, "How come my MD never told me to come to a Chiropractor?"

I said, "It's unfortunate, but medical doctors are not trained in matters of spinal subluxations, so they wouldn't know to detect and or correct it, let alone refer out to a Chiropractor."

She said, "I know I'm a bit far gone, but do you think you can do something for me?"

I said with a smile, "Yes." I put her on a care plan and adjusted her regularly.

We took progress films four months later and *she* had an *ah-ha moment* when she saw that the 42 degree curvature had reduced to 20 degrees. She looked at me and said, "Had I come to you five years ago, I could've avoided the four quadruple bypasses I had. I see that the area of curvature in my mid back supplies my heart."

Since improving her spinal alignment, Geraldine is now more active than ever. She plays bridge on a regular basis, gardens, moves her own furniture and cleans her own house.

Kurt

An *NHL* hockey player called my office and said his current Chiropractor in Minnesota told him to come see me, since I was one of the few Chiropractors in California using the technique he was used to (MC2). So when he was traded to the *Anaheim Ducks*, he drove forty-five miles three times a week from Tustin to Redondo Beach to get his adjustment.

He said, "Doc, I get beat up all the time on the ice, and the one thing that helps me to feel better and perform better is getting these specific adjustments." He then brought his pregnant wife for care. I worked with her all throughout her pregnancy, and when baby Cole was born I checked him as well. When the *Ducks* made it to the *Stanley Cup*, Kurt drove down to get his adjustment before he had to fly out to New Jersey to play in the finals. And when he landed home, he drove straight to my office before going back to *Disney Ice* to practice that same day. He did the same thing before and after the next games in the finals. This is one athlete who *got* Chiropractic. He correlated his peak performance with being unsubluxated.

Kelly

Kelly was trying to become pregnant for five years. She had two failed attempts with in-vetro fertilization. She almost lost her life during the last one due to adverse drug reactions. Every time she saw a baby she would think, "Why can't I have one?" She was in her early thirty's, 'healthy' for the most part, yet couldn't figure out why she couldn't become pregnant. Her mother Edith, already a patient of mine, recommended for Kelly to come to see me.

Edith said, "Maybe it's somehow related to your spine; why don't you get checked-out by Dr. G and see if Chiropractic can help." Kelly came in and I did a Chiropractic exam. Her scan clearly showed major subluxations in her upper cervical and lumbosacral regions. Her x-rays demonstrated a lumbar scoliosis with many postural abnormalities, and her scans looked like a lit up Christmas tree.

I put her on a care plan and four months later she came in with the biggest smile on her face announcing, "I'm pregnant!" Kelly had a beautiful baby girl, Evelyn; and of course I went to the hospital to give her first Chiropractic check up. Evelyn is now two years old and is as healthy as a Chiropractic child can be.

Tyson and Jacob

Gina brought her two sons into the office. Tyson was three and a half and Jacob was one and a half years old. Tyson has been through eighteen rounds of antibiotics since birth and Jacob has been through five rounds since birth. Since they had experienced so many reoccurring ear infections, their pediatrician said surgery was the next step. An adenoidectomy and tubes were eminent. The pediatrician did say she heard that Chiropractic may help, but she didn't know of anyone to refer to. Gina did her homework and found my office. The boys were very sickly and I was told they did not have more than 3 consecutive days of not being sick since being

being born. I did my Chiropractic exam and found multiple subluxations, and that their diet was in need of improvement.

After a month of Chiropractic care, both of the boys were free of ear infections and antibiotics. Gina was so amazed she said, "I'm going to write the President about this; I'm serious. He needs to know there are other options to help our children other than these horrible drugs; he needs to realize surgeries can be avoided." Neither Tyson nor Jacob have been on antibiotics since they started care. They are five and three now and are happy and healthy drug free boys.

Stepping Up

While I was having all these miracles happening in my office I had the honor of being asked to teach for the California Chiropractic Association (CCA) for technique relicensing hours. I gladly accepted the opportunity. I realized I had learned the art to delivering the goods in Chiropractic. I knew I had to share what I know. I integrated all three schools of thought (tonal, postural and segmental) plus cranial adjusting into a comprehensive approach of "*delivering da goods.*"

I was also privileged to speak on the stage at CalJam 2010. What a great gathering of like minded people. There's something to be said about mass consciousness vibrating at the same level: it is exhilarating and incredibly empowering.

Purpose

I realize I have been blessed with the best reason to get up out of bed each morning: to help other human beings live better lives. Chiropractic has afforded me this Soul Purpose. It is a noble profession to be proud of. No other profession on this planet has the type of impact on the human mind, body, and soul like Chiropractic. I may sound bias to an ignorant mind, and so it is our duty to tell the story.

All truths go through three stages. First it is ridiculed; second it is violently opposed; third it is accepted as self-evident.

~ *Schopenhauer*

- **Defining moments of truth.**
- **Use frustration as a catalyst for motivation.**
- **When the *student* is ready the teacher appears.**
- **When the *teacher* is ready the student appears.**
- **Recognize pivotal moments.**

The 'Checks' Of My Life
Dr. Justine Blainey-Broker

"You can't skate here. We'll have to add tampons to the first-aid kit!"

"You'll get hurt!"

"What are you doing here? You don't belong. This is a boy's hockey try-out!"

"No Girls on my ice!"

I could hear the sneering insults and whispers as I headed to the change room with my brother, Dave. He led the way and I followed, head down, trying not to let the things I heard sink in. We found a change room and, as I went to get on my underclothes (long johns etc.) in the bathroom, my bag was thrown out into the hall. They really didn't want me there and I knew I didn't fit in; but I wanted to. I am "that girl" who wanted to play hockey with the boys, to play higher level hockey with kids my own age, with body checking, more ice time, more games, and more coaching. I knew what I wanted, but I didn't realize the parents, administration and coaches would be so mean. I learned to hold my tears in, my head high, skate like the wind, and work harder than anyone else to prove myself and to *hit* the veterans.

In hindsight, my past challenges, the 'checks' of my life, have made the foundation for my character and my *backbone* today as a Chiropractor. I want to share with you the similarities between my fight for equality in sports and our current fight as Chiropractors in the health field.

It all started when my parents divorced and I wanted attention from my Dad. He watched Dave play hockey but not me doing my endless figure eights. I was jealous and I wanted to be recognized as valuable, talented and important.

A Chiropractor's emotions, too? You bet!

As the media attention grew over the oddity of a girl wanting to play boys' hockey, my 'friends' at school taunted me and refused to sit or have a locker beside me. I was shunned at school and at play to the same degree that I became 'famous' on every news channel at six o'clock. Across the country I was "That girl!" Classmates hissed insults; teachers slammed doors in my face and attempted to fail me because court attendance decreased school attendance. (I was in court battling for my rights to play hockey as a female.) Shocking graffiti was drawn on my locker. Hate mail, crank calls, and dangers in the streets, on the bus and on the subway followed. I was a hated *feminist* – the "F" word. I was called a butch and a slut who slept her way onto the team, and I was warned I'd never marry or have children. I had to leave friends behind just as wellness/subluxation Chiropractors have to separate themselves from sickness/pain based colleagues. I had to ignore insults and believe in my ideals, just as Chiropractors deal with taunting comments of not being "real" doctors and being "quacks!"

I was told I would ruin women's hockey. We all know that never happened! Now we have a well-supported, well-funded Gold Medal winning Canadian Olympic Women's Hockey Team – a team that toughened and tightened by playing in a male league. Similarly, wellness/subluxation Chiropractic has been designated as unworthy of serious consideration – Chiropractic is witchcraft! Women could never be strong enough, tough enough and would only get hurt playing with the boys, I was told.

Opinion is not truth, even majority opinion. Chiropractors are told pre-pay, wellness plans, adjustments without constant IFC or some modality will not "give" the patient enough for their money. Opinion is not truth and we Chiropractors must <u>never</u> stop believing in the true value of a life saving Chiropractic adjustment that does not need to be watered down with all the 'extras.'

My mother always said, "Sleep on it" when things seemed too tough and I was about to buckle under the pressures of being different, harassed and alienated. In the morning, I always affirmed that I was *not* a quitter; I was a proud feminist at ten years of age, just as I am a proud Chiropractor today.

I learned about Chiropractic at a young age because my brother suffered from mid-back pain. An MD referred us to Dr. Tom, our first Chiropractor, who diagnosed Dave within the first few minutes as having Scheuermann's Kyphosis Disease. Dave necessarily was adjusted regularly to help him breathe better, stop further degeneration, and play high level contact hockey, but my mother and I were only adjusted when we 'felt' something. We clearly did not 'get' the Chiropractic story. After suffering for years with asthma and migraines that hospitalized me and forced me to multiple Demerol shots after several bunches of handfuls of *Tylenol/Advil*, or anything I thought would help, I seriously sought an alternative and discovered more about the life saving benefits of Chiropractic adjustments. After a year of three times-a-week adjustments, my health gradually improved and all the while I continued to play hockey. I was asthma free and migraine free, and the strongest and healthiest I had ever been. Since, I am adjusted weekly – one or two times-a-week and have been for fifteen years!

After four plus years in court, from the Ontario Human Rights Commission to the Supreme Court of Canada and back to the Human Rights Commission, from ages ten to fifteen, I championed the change in the sports equality sections of the Ontario Human Rights code using the Canadian Charter. I finally won my court case in 1987. Hurray! I was 'legal!'

My brother and I tried out for the East Enders (MTHL 'A') along with eighty other hopefuls, and we both earned spots and signed player cards. I was so eager to call our coach and say, "Hi, I'm legal!" I had been practicing with the team, and cheering for Dave and our team for months during the court case.

I triumphantly called the coach and was told that he had given my spot away to a house leaguer – a lesser player – the night before, and there was not a player card left for me. I had two weeks to find a coach who would be brave enough to face his OHA masters and take the "first girl to play hockey with the boys legally."

"Fat chance," I thought. Tears and despair at the kitchen table. My brother, Dave, picked up the phone and said to the coach, "If there were a spot, could my sister have it?" The coach seemed to answer, "yes" because Dave responded without hesitation, "Then I quit – Justine can have my spot! She deserves to play and I will find another team."

"With two weeks remaining before the cut-off date?!" I thought. It was then that I realized the true value of support, of belief in the mission and who my real *team* was. Dave was willing to sacrifice the most important thing in his teenage life for the mission – belief in equality and in his sister's power. Are we willing to do that as Chiropractors for Chiropractic?

I was propelled to start developing *Justine's ways* of beating "the 'checks' of life." My approach certainly still helps me today as a wife, mother, sister, advocate, volunteer and Chiropractor.

Ask And You Shall Receive

The number one way to beat the 'checks' of life is to ask for help. At first, everybody seemed to say, "No Way!" Even my mom and dad. But Dave and I kept on asking. In my time of need, many feminists joined my family and lawyers. As Chiropractors, we need to gain strength by asking questions and by giving and receiving support to and from colleagues, in seminars, in person and on conference calls. We need to brainstorm our alliances and be loyal to each other and our ideals of Chiropractic. When we have calls of help to send in research, testimonials, and questionnaires to the OCA, CCO [our regulatory bodies and associations] and so on, we need to respond! We have a country and world to educate, and not only should we respond to requests, we should pro-actively search for opportunities to speak and educate.

Second, a way to beat the 'checks' of life is to realize that mistakes and challenges are part of normal growth. Not only was I not accepted by most of my male teammates, their parents, most of my own family and friends, but also women and female hockey players vehemently rejected me. It was a case of feminists against feminists and different beliefs about whether women's hockey should be pretty and all feminine versus rough and tough body checking like the boys.

Sound like Chiropractic? Wellness versus pain-based, low back specialists? You bet!

I learned to be excited for small achievements in my practice: the patient who slept better, who got sick less often, who could play sports more easily, who could lift the grandchildren or just loved to come for an adjustment but couldn't explain why. Each one was special. Each time I failed to handle an objection about adjustments and their true power, I learned a better way for the next time. I learned that I can handle and balance being a mom and a doctor and a volunteer if I trust and delegate more to team members. I can have more hours in the day for family as I maintain my personal health and passion. I don't have to do it all myself.

Third, I learned that innovation is truly just recreating or borrowing methods from those who walk before us. I was not the first girl to qualify for and want to play elite sport with the boys – Abby Hollyman and Gail Cummings had lead the way for me. We in Chiropractic have access to so many leaders and coaches. We can use and reuse their scripts, tested procedures, manuals and talks, handouts and paper-work. Leaders like Dr. Mike Reid, Dr. Liz Anderson–Peacock, Dr. Peter Amlinger, Dr. Sigafoose and so, so, so many more who have helped my practice double, triple, quadruple and more – not because of me, but because I and my team have used their tested and proven ways. Listen, learn, follow, copy and grow.

"Fake it until you make it," my brother would say to me. He used this line as he dated beautiful girls! Both on and off the ice I had to pretend I was tougher than I felt inside, espe-cially against the emotional abuse from friends, family and teachers. 'Fans' used to throw coffee or popcorn on me, and teachers refused to grant me access to work assignments and tests because I missed class to be in court. Certainly, Chiro-practors don't know all the answers and how to do every adjustment perfectly, in every situation, for example, our first day-old infant, our first patient with severe D.I.S.H. or R.A., or our first patient who asks us to help with incontinence or irritable bowel. We must not wait to know all the answers perfectly or to have attended every technique seminar avail-able. This is called "paralysis through analysis." Yes, keep on learning but Act! Go! Try! Believe! The adjustment works.

Sigafoose says, "Hit 'em with a brick and believe and it will be okay. Follow your innate." I believe this means trust your own healing powers and potential even if inside you're shaking a little.

Fourth, I talked and wrote to everybody I could. To beat the 'checks' we need to tell our story. Discrimination issues and equality issues with regard to access and funding are significantly improved now, but we still have a long way to go. Similarly, in Chiropractic we need to talk the "TIC" and share miracles: the miracle of Jake who had Bell's Palsy eliminated in one month of adjustments just before he went to college; the miracle of Joan who used to suffer from four migraines per day from being unable to work to being migraine/headache free and able to skate and dance again; the miracle of George with scoliosis and severe immobility returning to the golf course and off all medications; the miracle of eight year old Ashley missing school weekly because of headaches and stomach aches who is now feeling so great she joined the track team; and the miracle of Autistic Andre who used to come in wheelchair-bound, very loud and disruptive, now walking in with help to happily read books, high-five, give hugs and get adjusted! These are the miracles to share with everybody we know, to share hope and the Chiropractic message.

Fifth, to beat the 'checks' of life we need positive self-talk, meditation and gratefulness. My affirmations and goals are posted on my bathroom wall and mirror for me to review daily. As a family we do gratefulness bedtime routines. I know, for me, to handle the 'roughness' on the ice I needed to be physically and mentally prepared. Today, as a Chiropractor, my need for positive self-talk, meditation and gratefulness is ongoing. My day's 'homework' is always done before I start the next day (even if it means little to no sleep). I review the next day's patients to be ready for their specific needs and pray for their ongoing greatness and health.

Plan A, B, C. Enjoy the process.

I was cut from the Canadian Olympic Women's Hockey team hopefuls in tryouts having suffered a torn medial collateral ligament in my knee two weeks before national tryouts. Although hurt by my curtailed hockey dreams, I knew I also dreamed of being a great Chiropractor and helping others feel and live better. When one marketing event does not work for my practice, I simply move onto the next one. I have been taught to have multiple marketing plans and team plans, including daily handouts, internal and external talks, doctor's reports, anniversary reports, internal events, patient appreciation days, staff vision days, newspaper and radio advertisements, booths, flyers and much more! Many marketing events have failed to bring in new patients and we have had significant expenses, but I try to focus on the mission and dream of making a difference, to go fearlessly in my marketing and educational pursuits to find more potential patients to serve. I am there to help them – they just don't know it yet.

The sixth way to beat the 'checks' of life is to breath and be okay with having a negative moment. As so-called friends would come out of hiding to be on TV with me, I would just take a big breath and smile, because even pretend friends were better than no friends. When a patient goes "ahh," "ouch," moans, or negatively questions, I still take a deep breath. I remember that the challenges during my court case have strengthened women's hockey and female sport just as the stroke challenge and vaccination challenges have strengthened Chiropractic. Controversy means more people talking about what we do (positive or negative, the truth prevails either way). The more they notice us, the better for them and Chiropractic in the long run.

Patience...Perseverance

Remember the FOUR SW's: "Some will! Some won't! So what? Someone's waiting." The world is waiting and ready for us to share our miracles of health.

The seventh way to beat the 'checks' of life for me was to volunteer and show leadership. My brother and I started a "dress a girl" campaign in our high school to get young girls and teens an opportunity to try hockey. We wrote lists for the girls on how and in what order to put on their "newly-used-smelly" hockey equipment. I coached my peers on the ice and tutored them during and after school. In Chiropractic, I aim to give back and speak out about our mission and I am empowered as a person and as a Chiropractor when I do more, give more and serve more. After an educational lecture, I am always a better doctor the next day, for the talks always energize and stimulate me to my personal greater potential.

A Winning Attitude Trumps All

Eighth, a winning attitude is needed to beat the opposing, seemingly unbeatable 'checks' of life. As a hockey player, bruises and separated shoulders, injured knees and concussions meant "Game On!" I love to get sweaty, dirty and be in the game. All my best teams had great coaches. Thus, I believe in Chiropractic and life coaches for my team and me. I believe we were chosen to be Chiropractors by an innate power, but coaches and accountability partners help us reach our true potential, live up to the highest standard, play full-out and look forward to new 'checks.' Game On!

Today, I am a wife, mother, sister, daughter, friend, Chiropractor, advocate and volunteer, aiming to do my best. I know I can't be perfect and I can't please everybody, but I can try to be my best. My brother would tell me, "I can do it and so can you" when I would struggle with my slap shot or miss a hip-check. Today, as I observe other Chiropractic masters and 'have it out' with like-minded colleagues, I still repeat the phrase, "If they can do it, so can I." I am so thankful for my support team. Without them (Blake, Mom, Dad, Dave, my children, Margaret, and all my family, Dr. Mike, Kristine and many more), I would never have had the opportunity to serve as I do now. My mission is to make a difference. In my life and in Chiropractic, I need your help. Thank you.

Be brave, be powerful and be well!

- **Life prepares us in unusual ways.**
- **You CAN advocate for yourself, your patients, and your beliefs.**
- **Ask and you shall receive; it is okay to have a negative moment.**
- **Support is about giving and receiving.**
- **Stand up for fundamental rights.**
- **A winning attitude trumps all.**

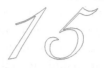

When Destiny Calls
Dr. Rose Lepien

"Why don't you apply for a job at the local Chiropractor," my mother-in-law asked?

I replied, "What's a Chiropractor?" As I walked into my first Chiropractic office in Red Bud, Illinois after a short interview, I was hired as a Chiropractic assistant; me: a twenty-three year old German girl, new to the United States, speaking broken English. With a smile on my face and an adventurous spirit in my heart, my journey in the wonderful world of Chiropractic began.

It was a marvelous experience being a Chiropractic assistant, learning patient care and all aspects of running an office. Coming from a small farm in Germany, with a degree in Home Economics and a minor in Physical Education, working in the field of Chiropractic was like 'coming home.' I found my calling.

Seek A Place And Space To Express Your Talents

In our journey through life we all seek to find that place and space where we can express our talents, while loving every moment of serving with fulfillment beyond measure. This I found in Chiropractic.

Then, life changed without warning. When my husband left my young son and me, when my Chiropractic employer left town due to a huge scandal resulting in the closing of his office, I found myself alone and without a job in this vast country.

My German family urged me to return to Germany. Had it not been for the burning love for this new found profession, and the recognition of my calling, I would have done so.

When one door closes, another one opens. A good friend hired me on his staff, resulting in a move to Port Huron, Michigan. Through my new position, my knowledge and experience as a Chiropractic assistant (CA) and office manager expanded and my love for this profession grew. I watched and experienced healing and Chiropractic miracles on a daily basis.

Life continued to unfold before my very eyes, as I followed my heart and married the "Love of my Life" – my employer, mentor and partner, twenty-five years my senior. We shared a joined passion for our profession, as well as a strong love for God and his Word. I am a living testimony that it is possible to be with your spouse 24/7, to create a dynamic life together, while raising children and stepchildren and dealing with the many challenges of daily life.

Each season in my life has taught me to live in the moment, to bloom where I was planted, and to mindfully walk through each 'room' of life with joyful anticipation and gratitude.

Show Excellent Stewardship

When we do well with little, showing excellent stewardship, when we give it our all every moment, God blesses us with bigger and greater endeavors. Patience certainly is a virtue that seldom goes unrewarded.

The following ten years were filled with opportunities to shine and serve as office manager, wife, and mother of my son and six stepchildren.

After my oldest stepdaughter graduated from Parker College's charter class of 1985, my destiny began to shift. A voice clearly spoke to me, "Go your way." As she entered our Lawton, Oklahoma Clinic as a Doctor of Chiropractic, my husband retired, and I enrolled at Parker College in 1988 at the age of thirty-eight. The Lord granted my wish to not go through Chiropractic College and menopause at the same time!

Wow, what an incredible journey, being in the womb of Chiropractic for three years: the learning, studying, testing, interacting and participating in student activities; the balancing of the student life and the personal life; the serving in various capacities in Student government and working closely with Dr. Jim Parker, founder of Parker Seminars and Parker College, and one of my most cherished mentors. Dr. Jim was totally dedicated, focused and fearless in taking his vision of Parker Seminar and Parker College worldwide. I was privileged to spend many hours with Dr. Jim, on campus, at the seminars and in his home. He asked me to be the student intern of Donna, his Lady, with direct instructions of how to treat her.

There are many stories to tell about Dr. Jim, but his dynamic character and his accomplishments tell them all. He was one of the true Chiropractic pioneers, giants and leaders, pushing our profession to the forefront, worldwide. In retrospect, spending time with Dr. Jim deepened my love for my college and our profession, and prepared me for later serving on the Board of Trustees at Parker College for nine years, four of which as Chairwomen of the Board.

Dr. Jim also recognized the uniqueness of female Doctors in the field of Chiropractic, and created the World Congress of Women Chiropractors (WCWC) in 1982, which had a strong chapter at Parker College. I recall my first WCWC meeting, standing up to share my story, as we still do at all WCWC meetings, my knees shaking. This special organization continues to connect and empower women Chiropractors around the world.

During my student life at Parker College, countless opportunities of serving presented themselves. I joyfully gave of my time, talents and resources, after receiving the message, "You shall pass this way but once, if there is anything that you can do, do it NOW, for you shall never pass this way again." This has become a concrete principle in my life, and oh, how I love it.

After graduation it was naturally-right to return to our Lawton practice. With passion I embraced this new role as a Doctor, and all the responsibilities entwined in it. My past experience as a Chiropractic assistant and office manager proved to be a valuable asset in the daily operations of the office, especially from a business aspect. Success in practice requires the duality of being an excellent Doctor and educator, as well as being business savvy. The second component is to attract and surround ourselves with a skilled and qualified team of employees that share our passion and vision. After thirty-seven years in this profession, I must confess that the staff issue is ongoing, forever changing, and at times challenging.

I have been very blessed with two great associate Doctors for twelve years, as well as three wonderful staff going on their thirteenth year. We became a dynamic family and a strong pillar in our community. Now that they have retired and/or moved on, I am back at hiring, orienting, training and educating new members of the team. New staff brings fresh perspectives, new energies, talents and interesting personalities, as well as continued opportunities to teach the wonders of Chiropractic.

Our office also offers a place for high school student interns attending the Chiropractic Assistant course at the local Vocational School. We plant a seed in every life we touch, but only God knows the harvest, so we just keep planting and growing.

On a fateful day in April 1997, my life changed drastically and permanently when my husband suffered a massive stroke. I watched as this brilliant man, my mentor, partner and best friend with a degree in Chiropractic, Internal Medicine, Metaphysics and Acupuncture became trapped in a crippled body. Total paralysis of his right side resulted. The loss of his ability to speak and communicate was the most difficult adjustment for both of us.

I recall a pivotal moment in the Emergency room, when his eyes begged me to come near to him, as he was on life support. Looking deep into my very soul, the question his mind was asking me was, "Should I fight to live, and will you stay with me to the end?" Holding his hand, with tears streaming down my face, this answer came over my lips: "I married you for better or for worse, for richer or for poorer, in sickness and in health, until death do us part." After taking a big sigh of relieve, he began to fight for his life, and our year and a half journey of a different kind of marriage began.

Balancing Demands

At a moments time, I found myself balancing the demands as a 24/7 caregiver, a mother, Doctor of a large clinic, now carrying all the responsibilities on my shoulders that I once shared with this handsome, experienced partner. We do not know our capabilities, until we travel the path, and God never gives us more to bear then we are able to carry. Life's experiences can make us bitter or better, our choice. I found myself reaching deep within my soul for strength, guidance and hope. It was a very lonely time.

Placing all my trust in God, he miraculously provided for a new associate to step into my practice, for patients to enter providing experience of dealing with a handicapped spouse, and for some of my stepchildren to step up to the plate and provide care when I was at the end of my rope.

The months that followed were the hardest, yet the most special months of my life.

My husband particularly enjoyed the days he accompanied me to our office. We treat our patients in a large, open room. It holds all the adjusting tables, therapy equipment and a few hospital beds, allowing interaction between the patients and staff. Watching me carrying on his life's mission, treating our patients, and visiting with them was the highlight of his week. I became very familiar with the world of the handicapped, and even ventured out onto road trips to Branson, Missouri, to Corpus Christy and to Michigan.

The most adventurous journey, however, was a trip to Germany to visit my family. I am still eternally grateful to the giant soldier, who bravely stepped in and assisted my husband in his wheelchair down a massive escalator at the Frankfurt airport. This trip turned out to be a divinely inspired and challenging one, as my mother unexpectedly passed away the third day of our visit. I miss her so, and the sense of loss is often overwhelming.

Transition

In September 1998, after a massive brain stem hemorrhage and three days in a coma, my husband passed. As I was holding on tight to his arm, setting him free, he took his last breath. At that very moment, when the monitor flat lined, I experienced a surge of great and powerful energy from his body into both of my hands. I was keenly aware of the breath taking fact that his life force, after separating from the tissue cells of his body, which was no longer capable of sustaining life, had entered into my hands. In the midst of this marvelous revelation, I perceived myself watching an 'instant movie.' Engulfed in this energy force, the movie entailed every thought, action, impression and experience of my husband's life. Then, slowly and gently, the energy with the attached information floated off into space.

In the twenty-five years of our marriage, this was the most powerful and lasting gift he ever gave me, the knowledge of the continuation of life after death, and the revelation that, who we are inside goes with us. Thank you, my love, for confirming the knowledge that we are all spiritual beings, having a human experience, for enriching my life in such a powerful way. Love never dies. Thank you for your repeated visits and words of guidance, I will see you on the other side.

In 2009 I published his latest book: *Life Before Life, The Journey of the Soul* (available on amazon.com). In the book he shares his spiritual and Christian believes, and reveals great discoveries resulting from many hypnotic sessions with patients and family members. The book has a unique style, and is as complex as he was. So he lives on, in this world and in the other.

Chiropractic Miracles

Treating patients for thirty-seven years, touching and healing not only the physical, but the emotional and spiritual body has been incredibly rewarding. As Doctors, we are all like magnets, attracting into our offices the people and conditions that resonate with our internal spirituality, talents and service attitude.

Since the Nervous System is the Master System, controlling all other systems, one must be totally open to incredible outcomes. The results of our treatment, the outcome of our interaction with our patients, are at times predictable, at times an awesome surprise. We are skilled and trained instruments, releasing the Innate Intelligence, which gives the body the power to heal itself.

Miracles happen every day, small and great, known and unknown. Through the years I have asked my patients to provide us with a written testimonial, and the book that compiles their stories gives hope and encouragement to countless others. Their testimonials touch lives and provide hope in our waiting room, in our treatment room, as well as on our website.

Allow me to share with you one such testimonial, the miracle story of Baby Nolan.

Nolan's mother and older brother were regular patients at my office; since receiving Chiropractic adjustments, the older brother has been relieved from severe reflux and leg cramps, and the mother was helped to deal with the stress and demands of family life. I treated the mother during the pregnancy of her twins, and did not see her until a few months after the twins were born. I vividly remember the day she entered the office with her twins, a boy and a girl, three months of age at the time, sharing the following history:

> When the twins were two weeks, old, the Doctors noticed that baby boy Nolan was not normal. He was not aware of his surroundings, never turned his head, was hardly eating, and did not move his left leg. Diagnosing him with dysplasia, he was put into a brace. The diagnosis of a mild stroke and Cerebral Palsy followed, with the recommendation to institutionalize him, since he was never going to have a normal life.

Tears streamed down the mothers face, as she reached out and handed me baby Nolan. Now, understand that I am a very experienced, confident Chiropractor, with great faith, confidence and belief in my skills, products, services and ideas. But at that very moment, as I was entrusted with the precious life of that little boy, my heart and thoughts went directly to God in prayer and petition for insight, guidance and direction. Following that inner guidance, after examining and observing Nolan, I concluded that he did not suffer from a stroke or from Cerebral Palsy. The upper cervical insult/subluxations from birth trauma were choking the life force from the brain to the body. I began to gently lay hands on Nolan, adjusting his little spine.

My heart leaped for joy, when later that evening a call came from the mother that Nolan had lifted his head and looked at her for the first time! As we continued adjusting him on a regular basis, we saw him change in front of our very eyes into a normal little boy. After two months of care, Nolan caught up to his little twin sister, and they continued on their journey of development and growth together, subluxation free, in a healthy and normal fashion.

A miracle had happened, a life had been changed and saved due to the power of a Chiropractic adjustment. This experience alone was worth all my education and hard work. My heart overflowed with gratitude and love. Practicing as a Doctor of Chiropractic is not about us, it is about being an instrument for God to touch and change lives. The monetary rewards are just an exchange for services rendered.

Then there was baby Sean, just six weeks old when his father brought him into my office. I have known his father since he was a young boy. Having worked in my Clinic years ago, he knew the power of adjustments.

At birth, Sean was addicted to drugs due to his mother's drug habits. After birth, he rarely slept or could keep any milk down, had difficulty coping with lights, noise or even touch by his parents. His body was in constant spasms. The entire family was in a panic. At the Children's hospital he was sedated and placed in isolation. He fought me with all his might when we began adjusting his little spine and applying cranial adjustments to his delicate little scull. His parents watched with amazement of the changes that followed:

> Relaxation of his muscles, decrease in his crying spells, he responded well to goats milk, his bowels started working normally, he started sleeping through the night and gaining weight. Today Sean carries his normal weight, smiles and responds to me. With anticipation he gets his adjustments on a once a month basis.

Then there was Mary, a lovely patient in her forties, with chronic female complaints. She was not able to afford, nor did she want to have the hysterectomy recommended by her medical doctor. An extensive Chiropractic and neurological examination with weight bearing X-Rays of the Lumbar spine revealed an advanced spinal curvature at the level of L2-L4, directly decreasing the nerve flow to her ovaries and uterus.

Regular adjustments, with stabilization of the curvature through therapy and a shoe lift provided Mary total recovery from all her symptoms without surgery and drugs.

My recommendation to choose Chiropractic first, medication second and surgery last continues to be heard throughout my office on a daily basis.

Amanda is a busy mother, wife and businesses partner to her husband. After the birth of her first child, she began to experience sharp pains in her lower back, tailbone and abdomen. She was medically evaluated with X-Rays of her kidneys, an ultrasound of her gallbladder, a colonoscopy, and endoscope followed laparoscopic surgery with a DNC, with no improvement in her symptoms. She was then diagnosed with 'Irritable Bowel Syndrome' and placed on medication to be taken for the rest of her life. She was referred to my office by her husband for a Chiropractic evaluation with weight bearing Lumbar x-rays.

After the very first adjustment, accompanied by stretching of her psoas muscle and balancing of the pelvic region, she was free of pain, after five years of suffering. She stopped taking her medication and is today enjoying her busy life subluxation free.

Brigitte is an accountant. She spends her days sitting at a computer, dealing on a continued basis with stressful situations. Tax season is the icing on the cake, and Brigitte's health and productivity depends on regular Chiropractic treatments.

She had a spinal fusion several years ago, but continues to suffer from chronic low back pain and sciatica. Being able to provide her relief from pain, as well as increase her quality of life and productivity has been a joy and a greatly rewarding experience. Brigitte is a committed Chiropractic patient for life.

Pat has suffered from recurring migraine headaches for years. She was literally told that it was "all in her head" and that she had to "learn to live with it," since no cause was found medically. After our evaluation it was revealed that she had fallen off a horse as a child, with injury to the upper cervical spine. She had been taking a great number of *Tylenol*, which started to damage her kidneys and stomach.

She was thrilled to learn about the connection of the C1-C3 (cervical plexus), supplying the nerve energy to the eyes, ears and head. She circled almost all the related symptoms on the nerve chart: headaches, irritability, high blood pressure, lack of concentration, sinus conditions, and fatigue.

After a series of cervical traction, trigger point therapy and spinal adjustments, with home stretches and nutritional therapy, her symptoms vanished and she began to live a normal life.

I hear many patients report that they were not aware of how poorly they felt, until they started experiencing quality of health after the adjustments. Today Pat tells everyone "You don't have to live with headaches."

I am thrilled to share and teach the power of a Chiropractic adjustment everywhere I go. The Chiropractic profession in this country celebrated its 110th anniversary, but the benefits of an adjustment remain the best-kept secret in town. Statistics indicate that only 15-20 percent of our entire population is under Chiropractic care. Hundreds of opportunities arise every day as we are planted firmly in our communities and towns. I accept every invitation to give a health related talk at local churches and non-profit organizations, to participate in health fairs, career days at the schools, and give my time to provide sports physicals for the Salvation Army Boys & Girl's Club.

My profession has afforded me to travel to Columbia, South America and to Rio, Brazil for the Pan American Olympics, adjusting athletes to assure maximum performance in their disciplines. My travels in Chiropractic have also lead me to Australia, Canada, Portugal, Italy and Germany. Everywhere I go, there are spines!! The world is hungry for the powerful message of hope that Chiropractic delivers, while searching for wellness and excellence in body, mind and spirit. A life of high quality is not achievable with a sick nervous system.

My patients are empowered to go and take the Chiropractic message into their circle of life, with the knowledge that lives can be saved and changed if they reach out and speak up. Please help us spread the message, tell the story, and ask the question: "Have you been adjusted lately."

We have all been called to instill into our patients and friends the value of exceptional health and wellness, the role that Chiropractic plays, as well as the role their choices play in the quality of their lives. The United States has the most modern medical facilities, tests and treatments available and is the richest Nation on this planet. Sadly enough, it also has the sickest population of all the countries in this world! We are Chiropractic warriors, called to live and to teach the Chiropractic message to all people, at all times.

- **Seek place and space to express your talents.**
- **Show excellent stewardship.**
- **Transition is part of the natural flow.**
- **Have you been adjusted lately?**
- **Balancing demands – ask for help.**

Conceive, Believe, Achieve
Dr. Lezlee P. Detzler

When you have passion for something in life, anything is possible. Limitations can be overcome. Barriers are eliminated. Opportunities abound. My passion is Chiropractic. From an early age, I observed and learned from my parents, who had their own business that you had to work hard to achieve success. It was sort of a "Have-Do-Be" formula. If you wanted to "have" something you "did" what it took to get it and then you could "be" happy and successful because of it. Initially, I was coming from a place of "having" the things that defined success for me – my own busy Chiropractic office, student debts repaid, and respect in the community and of my colleagues; the list went on and on. I came out of school with this burning desire and passion to be an accomplished Chiropractor - I thought I had it all figured out. However, through my own experience, frustration and intense reflection, I later discovered I had the formula reversed. It is actually "Be – Do – Have." I must first "be" the person I want to be, before "doing" the things I need to do in order to "have" what I want, as long as they were aligned with my passions. This allowed my values and true self to shine through, and in turn to "have" success, within the parameters I defined.

My First Chiropractic Experience

> Throughout the vastness of our Universe, there is an abso-
> lute intelligent order that exits... this intelligent order is
> run by an all-pervading energy that encompasses and con-
> trols everything from the movements of the planet, and the
> tides of our oceans, to the changing of the seasons and
> even the activities of the human body.
> ~ *Michael Talbot,* author of *The Holographic Universe*

It is said that adversity can be a teacher. My life is no exception to that rule. At the age of thirteen, I was plagued with
bouts of head pain that began to increase in frequency and
severity. The head pain became so relentless that I started
missing days at a time from school, which put graduating
from Grade 8 in jeopardy. My mother initially took me to a
medical doctor and then to numerous specialists to determine the cause of my head pain. The doctors thought I might
have a brain tumor, so a CAT scan was performed. When the
scan came back negative and they couldn't find any cause for
the extreme head pain, they suggested to my mother that it
must be psychosomatic; it was all in my 'head.'

Fortunately, my mother knew there was no way I would
fake head pain as an excuse to miss school. As a last resort,
my mother travelled thirty miles from our hometown to take
me to a Chiropractor. The Chiropractor asked my mother a
lot of questions, performed a spinal examination and took
some x-rays of my spine and neck. He diagnosed me as having a scoliosis and multiple vertebral subluxations. It was the
Chiropractors' clinical opinion that I was suffering from migraines. He was highly suspect the vertebral subluxations
and scoliosis were contributing to the migraines. He explained that Chiropractic is a unique health care field
dedicated to the detection, correction and prevention of vertebral subluxations in order to eliminate spinal nerve
interference which adversely affects one's health. When I

questioned my Chiropractor as to how the vertebra become subluxated, he responded that the primary cause of subluxations is stress – physical, chemical, emotional and/or mental. He said a combination of all of these stressors overwhelms the body's natural ability to adapt and decreases the body's resilience and coping mechanisms. By correcting vertebral subluxations, his goal was to normalize function, by removing a significant impediment to nature's inborn ability to heal. Health, then, is truly an inside-out phenomenon, not an outside-in application. He assured my mother that regardless of my symptoms, the vertebral subluxations of my spine warranted the need to be under Chiropractic care.

We learned that Chiropractic is a blend of art, science and philosophy, with a strong underlying belief that "the power that made the body, heals the body," often referred to as healing from "above, down, or inside out." This power that the human body has is what Chiropractor's term "Innate Intelligence" or "Life Force" - an inner wisdom or an inborn Intelligence emanating within every cell of the body.

The Chiropractor asked if I ever wondered how our heart beats from the day we are born until the day we die, or when you cut yourself how the body knows how to heal itself. He explained that this innate intelligence uses the brain and nerve system to control and maintain the health of the body. He added that the body is a self-healing, self-regulating organism and that all bodily functions in a human being are under the direction of the nervous system. Chiropractors were not the only ones purporting this, as Andrew Weil, Medical Doctor said, "Healing comes from inside, not outside..."

He contended that vertebral subluxations, by interfering with the central nervous system, impedes the body's normal function, reducing its ability to self-regulate, adapt, and heal, and this affects our overall health.

During one of my visits to his office, I remember reading a poster on his wall that quoted Thomas Edison: "The doctor of the future will give no medicine, but will interest his patients in the care of the human frame, in diet and in the cause and prevention of disease." I knew from that moment forward I was onto something really big with Chiropractic. I felt a connection with the Chiropractic Philosophy, and most importantly at the time, was so grateful there was hope that someone could help me. After the first three months of receiving Chiropractic care, my life changed. The intensity, duration and frequency of my migraines were all dramatically reduced. I remember with each visit to the Chiropractor, he would share more information regarding the nervous system telling me how it is responsible for coordinating the function of every cell, tissue and organ in the body in order for the body to function optimally. He explained to me how the Vertebral Subluxation Complex (VSC) causes interference with the nervous system and that Chiropractic is the only healing science responsible for locating and correcting subluxations via the Chiropractic adjustment, thereby restoring the body's ability to heal itself.

From this point forward, I was incredibly fascinated by the 'Chiropractic adjustment' and the miraculous improvements it had on my migraines. I became captivated with the human body and the nervous system; it was mind boggling to think of the degree of precision and perfection in which the body functioned in spite of our efforts to the contrary. Our innate intelligence has our heart beat one hundred thousand times each day. Our veins and arteries would stretch approximately twelve thousand miles if laid out in a line. An average newborn baby starts with the unification of only two cells and within nine months proliferates to six billion cells in the form of organs, tissues, and bones. We wear out approximately ten million red blood cells each second, but our innate intelligence (life force) is constantly replacing them with new ones. There are more than six hundred muscles in our body – many of them working as a team. In some ways it was a blessing to be plagued with migraines at a young age.

These magnificent revelations captured my interest and solidified my desire to become a Chiropractor at the age of thirteen. Now I'm in my twenty-sixth year as a chiropractor and have never looked back.

Conceive, Believe, Achieve

> The only place where dreams are impossible is in your own mind.
> ~ *Emalie*

One of the greatest positive motivators of all time, Napoleon Hill said, "What the mind can conceive and believe, it can achieve," and don't I know it. I'm sure most people can empathize when I say that at times in my life I doubted my abilities. I was met with several obstacles to becoming a Chiropractor, and they were mostly self-imposed. Although it did not always feel like an easy career path, I persisted because there was nothing else I wanted more, than to be a Chiropractor.

During my undergraduate years, one of my university professors expressed concern I would never pass his human kinesiology course and suggested I drop the course and change programs. His comments were a blow to my self-confidence. I started to doubt my academic abilities. I considered quitting university all together, and at one point returned home to my parent's house, deflated, where I stayed for nearly a week.

As the Universe would have it, persistence and determination were also part of my innate intelligence and so, with their encouragement, I dug my heels in and returned to university. I decided I would not give in to meeting the core requirements needed to gain entrance into Chiropractic College.

Once accepted, here again arose the doubt and fear. At about the sixth week into my courses, I was completely lost in my biochemistry class. I felt I had stepped in over my head and that the class was beyond my educational abilities. Over that Thanksgiving weekend, I told my family I was quitting yet again. They reminded me that becoming a Chiropractor was all I ever talked about.

After their much-needed pep talks and support, I was able to re-focus and return to school. I remembered something important about that weekend that I now tell my nieces and nephews, "If you want something bad enough and are disciplined and believe in yourself, you can achieve anything you want to in life."

I packed up, taking my own advice and the words of Napoleon Hill, and went back to Chiropractic College. I was able to realize the great gift that was my support system, and continued to utilize it. Again, as the Universe acknowledged my absolute commitment and belief in this decision, another support system landed in my lap. One of my fellow students majoring in biochemistry noticed my difficulty with the course and offered to tutor me, and the rest was history. I graduated four years later cum laude with honors.

After graduation, I spent a year as an Associate learning from a seasoned Chiropractor. I was young and impressionable and thought that his way must be the 'right' way and I should follow his same methods. He was clearly successful in his practice, and appeared to have everything he desired out of life. I adopted his methods into my own budding practice and quickly learned how important it is to find your own style, pace, method, environment, and more importantly to be authentic, centered and balanced. I certainly benefited from his mentoring and the wisdom of others along the way; however, none of my initial decisions were original to me.

My head was full of facts, stats and all kinds of data. I had more Chiropractic knowledge than the Canadian army had artillery. I assumed I had all the tools I needed to handle the barrage of new patients that were going to come crashing down my doors. What a humbling experience.

First, the potential new patients didn't even know who I was or where I was, in order to come crashing down my door. I had all this knowledge and a burning passion to heal the world, but patients seemed unclear after my explanation of Chiropractic. I learned I was coming across as either too scientific or too philosophical, as I'm sure, many new graduates do. I had spent six plus years in post-secondary education environments relating to textbooks, professors and colleagues, and very little time with 'real' patients. Yes, I had accumulated a lot of knowledge, but had very little experience relating that knowledge to other people. I also had an undeveloped concept or knowing of 'self.'

My primary focus after graduation was to build a large Chiropractic practice (for many reasons). First and foremost, I had huge debts to pay off. I also craved the respect and status that came with being a 'Doctor' through having my own busy clinic, house, and car among other things. I wanted to get all of the external things right - my staff, the marketing system, the community, the patients, the billing – all of which had to do with what was outside of me. If I'm being honest, I wasn't necessarily aware that anything other than those factors even existed. I knew I didn't *love* all of the things that my mentor was doing in his office, but if his procedures could be improved upon, that would bring me fulfillment and success.

So I did not pay much attention to the energy or space around me or inside of me to define who I was as a person (I will elaborate on shortly). As an Associate, I realized it was a good place to start my journey as a Chiropractor. I recommend that Chiropractors who are just entering the profession (as well as seasoned practitioners) use coaches or mentors. Those critical partnerships can and should be formed with people who possess like-minded values and beliefs. It was largely because of the fundamentals I learned in that great mentorship that I was able to develop and maintain a busy practice for many years.

My Transformation

Always be a first-rate version of yourself, instead of a second-rate version of somebody else.
~ *Judy Garland*

One of the most significant lessons I learned as a Chiropractor is that success in any area of your life does not come from the outside of you – what you "have" or "do" such as your office location, adjusting technique, office procedures, scripts, staff, town or city. It comes from the inside of you - who you are or *be*, your passions, values, beliefs, level of certainty, enthusiasm and thoughts, just to name a few. In my first few years in practice, I was a human *doing*, not a human *being*. Thank goodness I learned over time that "thoughts become things" and that some of my previous thoughts held me back from blossoming into a human *being*, and kept me in a place as a human *doing* for years.

After being an associate Chiropractor for one year, I moved on to open my own clinic. I was set on mirroring my first mentor's method for success, and although I was able to establish a respectable practice, my practice was not functioning as smoothly as my mentors; it required a lot more hours and hard work. At times I was very frustrated, as I wasn't achieving my goals. I followed all of my earlier gurus' suggestions. I had written out my one, two, five and ten year goals that were S.M.A.R.T. (specific, measurable, attainable, realistic with a time frame). I had a mission statement for my office; I used daily affirmations. I had my favorite inspirational quotes hanging throughout my office; I thought I was 'doing' it all 'right' to 'have' it all, in order to 'be' what I considered successful, happy and fulfilled.

Approximately four years later my Chiropractic practice

reached a plateau and my energy was at an all time low. I knew I had to do something different.

I decided to seek new ideas by attending Chiropractic seminars. I became a seminar junky. I attended dozens of workshops across North America. I wanted a large successful practice so desperately that I was chasing it in every book and speaker I could find. I spent all weekend listening to successful Chiropractors tell their story and share what was working for them. I returned to the office Monday mornings with a briefcase full of new office forms and procedures. I changed the office hours; incorporate more staff meetings, and a myriad of other things.

I was *high* from the seminar hype of the weekend, armed with new ideas and material to take my practice to the next level. And yes, the practice would rise to a new level for a few months; however, it was not sustainable. So, off I went four or five months later to another seminar. My 'Chiropractic seminar fixes' drove my staff crazy; they dreaded the post-seminar Monday mornings.

It seemed I was constantly striving in practice, not thriving (synergy with my surroundings). One evening, around eleven, after writing up my last x-ray report for the night, not yet having had my dinner, I put my head in my hands and cried. I thought to myself, "I can't keep doing this. I am exhausted, I have no balance or fun in my life, I am unhappy and unfulfilled – I AM BURNING OUT." It was not how I imagined my life as a Chiropractor, working sixty to eighty hours, six days a week, my clinic hours all over the map, my staff improperly trained, I was seeing approximately two hundred patients per week, had very little time to take care of my own needs, minimal time for family, and no holidays.

As the Universe would have it, a colleague and very good friend mentioned to me, numerous times, a Practice Management Group, Carter Associates. My colleague had been a part of this group for two years and found them to be different from the others he had attended. He said it altered who he was inside, which in turn revolutionized his practice. Seeing the success and fulfillment in his life, I took his advice and committed to the Carter Program for a four year term. It was a significant commitment of time and money, neither of which I had a lot. Although I could not have known this at the time, it became the most significant source of transformation in my life. My decision for joining the program was twofold: (1) to decrease the stress in my life, and (2) to operate a successful practice without increasing the number of patients in my office. It was my belief at the time that I could not possibly see any more patients during the hours my clinic was operating.

From my first day as a Chiropractor, I have always had passion, certainty and enthusiasm for what I "DO" as a Chiropractor. It was during my initial years in practice, while attending Parker Seminars, I was introduced to the concept of having 'faith, confidence and belief' (FCB) in your 'product, service and idea' (PSI) – this is what enabled me to create an average practice. It was during my four years in Carter Associates that I developed this sense of knowing and conviction for Chiropractic from a place inside of me - the "BE", with absolute certainty, passion and enthusiasm. It was then that my Chiropractic practice and life skyrocketed to a new level.

Carter Associates program was three fold for me: (1) who I "BE," (2) creating an office space to support who I "BE" and, (3) reinforcing my certainty and conviction for Chiropractic and the incredible innate ability of the body to heal itself. Initially, Dr. Carter addressed who I was 'being' as a Chiropractor, the inside of the practice and the practitioner. He had me revisit my values and beliefs and identify what motivated, inspired, and fulfilled me from the inside out. Until this point in my life I was a "HAVE-DO-BE" Chiropractor. Throughout the next four years I transformed to a "BE-DO-HAVE" Chiropractor. I finally discovered how I wanted to 'be' as a Chiropractor versus what I wanted to 'have'. The transformation looked something like this. I went from:

- Making my Chiropractic practice about me, *to* making it about my patients;
- Selling Chiropractic, *to* teaching/educating patients about Chiropractic;
- Telling/advising patients what to do, *to* supporting them in their health care decisions;
- "Should and have," *to* "choose to;"
- Using confrontation with patients regarding their Chiropractic care, *to* 'care-frontation' (confronting with compassion, care and concern);
- Giving adjustments to patients, *to* sharing an adjustment with patients from my heart to theirs
- From conditional love for my patients, *to* unconditional love;
- An unbalanced life (all work), *to* a more balanced life;
- Being competitive in the health care industry, *to* being collaborative;
- Telling the patients what they wanted to hear (inauthentic), *to* telling them the truth about the vertebral subluxation and its consequences to their overall health and wellbeing.

So what brought on these transformations? Well, part of the Carter Program consisted of several experiential weekend workshops and I mean *experiential*. Our mind can be our greatest strength/support or our greatest weakness/critic. Henry Ford said, "Whether you think you can or think you can't, you're right." I had so many limiting beliefs around my capabilities and potential, in regard to my Chiropractic practice. Let me share with you one particular experiential workshop regarding the power of my mind that proved to be very insightful. Think about the potential of taking your mind to the next level by stretching yourself physically, to a level you wouldn't think possible. I consented to participate in a one hundred and fifty foot fire walk on red-hot coals. The instructor told us this particular fire walk was exactly one hundred and fifty feet long, so I focused at precisely one hundred and fifty feet. I walked the entire length of this fire walk with no burns until the last five feet. I lost my focus and boy, did I burn my feet.

That night as we were debriefing the event, the instructor informed me that I had an incredible power of focus with extreme precision. I was confused, if this were true, then why did I burn my feet on the last five feet of the fire walk? He replied, "We made a mistake, the fire walk was one hundred and fifty-five feet." Once I deemed I had completed one hundred and fifty feet, my body was not able to resist the red-hot coals any longer. My state of mind determined my body's ability to resist the forces around it. From this (painful) experience, I learned that I will achieve exactly what I set out to do in my mind, and no more than that - a life changing lesson. I decided to shoot for the moon from that point forward, because I knew I would always at least hit the stars.

This was the beginning of the transformation in myself and in my Chiropractic practice. The practice was no longer about me (my debts, my success, my ego); it became about the patients, their successes and life changing events with Chiropractic care. I was seeing lives transform through the power of the Chiropractic adjustment. Patients described having improved thinking and clarity; they described their life as happier and healthier. They became aware that Chiropractic was so much more than just the treatment and relief of pain. I went from using a cornucopia of fluid office procedures to a customized system of solid procedures where all the staff were cross-trained and 100 percent competent.

I discovered it is important to find out what works for you in your practice and do it to the best of your ability. I discovered it is best to delegate to staff anything you are doing in your office that draws your energy away from what you love to do. I brought balance into my life by doing this and with this balance I was happier. I reduced my hours, attended more seminars, spent more time with colleagues, my partner, my family and friends and the outdoors. I created a life outside of my practice, and this only contributed to the success within my practice and with my patients. When all of the logistics of my office became aligned with my passion and values, it was then I took my practice and life to a new level.

So now I live my life as advised by Dr. John Demartini, who said, "Do what you love and love what you do, and you will never work a day in your life."

Miracles And Marvels

> There are only two ways to live your life. One is as though nothing is a miracle. The other is as though everything is a miracle.
> ~ *Albert Einstein*

During my ten years in private practice, many Chiropractic miracles occurred. I remember one patient who had been seeing me for some time. One day, she arrived for her regular adjustment and was very upset. She described how it just broke her heart to see her grandson struggle so terribly at school; he was in Grade 4 but reading at a Grade 2 level. His grandmother tried to help him, but he resisted, saying he, "hated reading." She was convinced the concussion he suffered two years earlier while playing hockey had something to do with his poor reading ability and his personality change.

Prior to the hockey injury she described her grandson as full of life, energetic, happy, confident and very healthy prior to the hockey injury. After the concussion he had very little drive or determination, his hockey abilities deteriorated, and he was continually coming down with ear, nose, and throat infections. An examination and x-ray of her grandson revealed a reverse curvature in his neck and multiple vertebral subluxations.

Within eight months of starting Chiropractic care his reading went from a Grade 2 to Grade 4 level. His self-esteem soared, as did his energy and health. His grandmother expressed sincere gratitude for how Chiropractic changed his life; she felt like she had her grandson back again. His parents were so astonished and thankful at the change in their son they too became patients at the clinic.

Another illustration of the power of Chiropractic involves a very special lady who became a patient of mine during my second year in practice. A patient of mine asked if I'd see a friend of hers who had multiple sclerosis (MS) so severe that she was now bedridden. I did an examination of her at her house and diagnosed multiple vertebral subluxations. I explained to her that I was not treating her MS; however the multiple subluxations in her spine were causing nerve interference and hindering her own body's healing ability. We began Chiropractic adjustments at her home.

During one of my Chiropractic visits to her house she told me that one of her greatest passions was dancing and how she has never lost hope that one day she would be able to dance again. After months of Chiropractic home visits, she reached a point in her healing where she was able to come to the office with assistance. Eventually she was able to bring herself to the office; she was ecstatic. I will never forget the day she walked into my office beaming with energy, sporting the broadest smile I had ever seen on her face. She said to me, "You'll never guess what.... I danced again; all night long."

It brought tears to both her eyes and mine. She gave me the biggest hug. Chiropractic changed her life, and mine.

Locum-In-Motion

The greatest danger for most of us is not that our aim is too high and we miss it, but that it is too low and we reach it.

~ *Michelangelo*

When I graduated from Chiropractic College I had a twenty-year plan with very specific goals and markers. After only ten years in practice I realized I arrived at this twenty-year mark, ten years earlier than anticipated. One of my goals at my twenty-year mark was to practice as a locum Chiropractor. So it was now time to re-evaluate my situation and focus on the next chapter in my life. With much debate, heartache and conviction, I sold my practice. I wasn't sure if I was walking away from something or towards something else, but knew it was time for change. I bought a one year, one-way ticket that would take me around the world. My first long-term stop was New Zealand; feeling somewhat exhilarated, exhausted and inspired, I performed my first Chiropractic locum. For almost 25 years my identity had been attached to becoming and being a Chiropractor. I felt like I had lost part of who I was when I left my Chiropractic practice. Having my practice was partly how I identified myself. Needless to say I was very happy to jump back into Chiropractic, and adjust patients, after my sabbatical. Although the offices, procedures and protocols varied in New Zealand, the Chiropractic Principles and philosophy were the same world wide.

Upon my return to Canada after one year abroad, I decided to continue my locum work. Becoming a locum seemed like the best of many worlds for me. I was able to continue being part of the Chiropractic community and doing what I loved to do – adjust patients, educate about the power of the body's innate ability to heal, and share Chiropractor success stories. Being a Chiropractor is so much more than treating someone's pain or symptoms; it is about enhancing a patient's overall health and well-being. I have seen Chiropractic have an impact on all seven areas of people's lives – mental, social, physical, family, financial, professional and spiritual. Also, as a locum Chiropractor, I can be fully present with a patient and let them know I hear them and I care. As a locum Chiropractor, I contend a successful practice is not solely contingent on the place (city/province/ country), the economy, the office procedures, the staff or the technique. As I have worked in numerous successful Chiropractic offices throughout Ontario and in other countries, it is apparent the aforementioned variables differed from office to office while each practice was still successful. The one common denominator was who the Chiropractor was *being*.

I'd like to share a heartfelt story about a young boy I had the privilege of seeing as a locum Chiropractor. His mother brought him in to see me as a new patient when he was approximately eight years old. I'll never forget his manner - a lifeless little boy with no self-esteem, no zest for life. He made no eye contact with me nor did he answer any of my questions. Needless to say he was not the typical eight-year-old boy. His mother brought him in for chronic leg pains that were apparently hindering his ability to partake in sports. She described him as being inactive and quite withdrawn. Throughout the consultation the rest of the story unfolded – he was a bed wetter since age four. This boy's life was being severely limited. He was petrified to attend sleepovers and participate in other activities for fear of having a bed wetting experience; it would have been humiliating for him had his peers found out. His mother said he felt like an outcast - felt that something was wrong with him. This boy had multiple subluxations throughout his spine, especially in his low back. I explained to his mother that these subluxations could be contributing to his symptoms and that it was important to get his spine and nervous system functioning at its optimum level by commencing Chiropractic care. Seeing a Chiropractor was their last hope, as the mother was informed by the doctors all they could do was wait until her son eventually 'grew out of' his disorders. I also suggested to his mother to enroll him in a martial arts program to help boost his self-esteem. She was eager to comply.

One year later, when I was back at the same office as a locum, the same boy was scheduled to see me. When I walked into the room, my jaw dropped. I saw a child with a sparkle in his eye. He made eye contact with me. I could see the zest for life that was previously missing and a huge amount of confidence and vitality emanated from him. He was thrilled to tell me that his leg pain had resolved and he was on his fourth belt in karate. His mother said Chiropractic care gave him his life back. "We never know how far reaching something we may think, say or do today, will affect the lives of millions tomorrow," said B.J. Palmer. In that moment I was blessed with seeing the direct result of my being a Chiropractor – a gift I am forever grateful for. I am reminded almost daily how fortunate I am to be a part of such a life changing profession, and for the lives we are blessed to touch and affect.

Adversity Happens For A Reason

> Your purpose may forever remain obscure to you, but you can rest assured that you're fulfilling your destiny.
> *~ Buckminster Fuller*

During my years in practice, if a patient discontinued care I asked myself what could I have done better for the patient or what didn't I do that I could have. When my practice waxed and waned with its ups and downs, I sometimes doubted my abilities as a Chiropractor. It was important for me to remember not all patients are going to be a perfect fit for my office, nor me a perfect fit for them. During those times it was also important for me to remember all the wins and miracles over the course of my career.

At a previous point in my life I achieved everything I set out to achieve in practice in a timeframe ten years sooner than expected. I started to drift around and think about what I needed to "do" with my life – asking am I doing enough, am I contributing enough.

During a simple stretch in bed early one morning, I experienced an excruciating pain in my neck and arm that radiated down to my fingers. At first I thought I'd been shot in the neck with a bullet from outside my window, but then I realized I had damaged a disc in my neck. Within a few days it was confirmed by an MRI that I had an acute disc herniation at C6 and C7. I spent the next three months flat on my back, immobilized and in extreme pain. I saw two neurologists and received conflicting opinions; one said I must get surgery immediately to prevent further damage, and the other said I had nothing to lose by waiting a year to see what happens. These two conflicting opinions gave me a great deal of compassion for what some of my previous patients had gone through. I was experiencing first hand how terrifying it can be when in such extreme pain and not knowing which way to turn.

For months, I had to lie perfectly still on my back as it was incredibly painful to sit with the weight of gravity on my head. I couldn't walk, as with each step the pain increased in my neck and radiated into my arm; it was unbearable. The neurosurgeon who suggested immediate neck surgery gave me a grave prognosis; a 50 percent possibility I might lose some of the function of my arm or hand. The only thing I ever wanted to be was a Chiropractor, and I started to believe I would never practice again. One of my best friends, a colleague of mine came to my house to adjust me daily. Within three months, I was able to sit up with considerably less pain. I was soon able to walk for five minutes at a time.

With persistent, consistent Chiropractic care, some intermittent acupuncture for pain control, and no drug intervention at all, I was able to return to work as a Chiropractor eight months later. The Universe definitely stopped me in my tracks and I had a full three months to go from "doing" to "being." I had a lot of time to reflect and think about where my life might be heading next. I realized how fragile life is. I always thought of myself as completely healthy. If it hadn't been for my incredible conviction for Chiropractic and the body's ability to heal itself, I am not sure I would have recovered. To this day, I still have a disc (cervical) herniation that occasionally flares up. When I listen to my body and practice self-care, I am still able to practice part-time and fulfill my passion to support other Chiropractor's as a locum. I am much more cognizant of my body – it tells me when I am doing too much or not enough. This eight month hiatus in my career allowed me to revisit my passions and goals. Chiropractic was still tops on my list of passions. At this time, I also recommitted myself to my own health, fitness and spiritual wealth.

Out Of Africa

> People may not remember exactly what you did, or what you said, but they will always remember how you made them feel.
> ~ *Maya Angelou*

I had the privilege of doing volunteer Chiropractic at a non-profit organization facility in Jambiani, Tanzania, East Africa known as Hands Across Borders. This facility provided the opportunity of complimentary Chiropractic care to those people in need on the island and from the mainland of Africa. I spent one month in Jambiani and witnessed how the power of faith and trust in Chiropractic changed these people's lives. Although they understood very little as to what Chiropractic was, they knew through others testimonials and their own experiences that Chiropractic helped their body heal and enhanced their life. Some of the locals came to the clinic because of musculo-skeletal problems and others sought Chiropractic adjustments because they just had an inside knowing that it was good for them. Given the language barrier, often the fewer words you said the more they understood. It felt like I was treating them from my heart to theirs. Even though we had an interpreter, the interpretations were from Swahili to English. The faith and confidence people had in what we did was powerful.

One of the most interesting and moving stories for me was a woman who presented to our clinic, recently having suffered a stroke. She lost most of the function on the left side of her body and her speech was also somewhat impaired. Within a few days after her stroke, she was brought from the major city Stone Town, to our clinic in Jambiani. By the time I arrived for my one-month assignment, she had already been through one week of Chiropractic care after her stroke. Never in my 20 years of Chiropractic practice had I adjusted a patient so recently after suffering a stroke. To say the least, I was somewhat apprehensive to adjust her neck. It was truly amazing, the rapidity of healing and transformation that occurred with this lady in one month with Chiropractic care. Despite her desperate condition, she had a strong faith and trust in Chiropractic; it should not have surprised me the miracle she was experiencing. It brought tears to my eyes to witness her profound improvement from one visit to the next.

Joy And Fulfillment

Life is not measured by the number of breaths we take, but by the moments that take our breath away.
~ *Hilary Cooper*

We all have something in our life that empowers us, whether it is a person, place, activity or thing. When you connect with that something you feel like all is right in the world. You have purpose, you are touching others and you are gloriously happy. For me that is obviously Chiropractic... but it happens in so many other related ways as well. I LOVE inspiring and empowering patients to live a healthy and extraordinary life. I LOVE to sit down and educate patients about the Chiropractic story and how it can literally change their lives. And then there is the regular office visit – patients knowing I am truly hearing and appreciating them (remember that people do business with people they know, like and trust), being witness to patients' lives changing via the power of the adjustment – the miracles of Chiropractic. Hearing patients say, "That is the best examination I have ever had" or "You are the first doctor who has heard what I am saying." I LOVE being able to give hope to someone who is feeling defeated; hope that someone can help them; that I can help them. I LOVE telling new patients that extraordinary health isn't expensive, and two months later them telling me I was right, it's priceless.

Despite my diligent work ethic with my career and determination for success, family has always been a priority for me. My most faithful patient has been coming to me for care since I graduated from college. Talk about faith, confidence and belief in Chiropractic, this woman traveled 45 minutes for 25 years (from the age of 65 to 90), to receive regular spinal adjustments. For someone who, until recently, had an active lifestyle and could be found playing cards, at church, or visiting her family, she always made time for her commitment to Chiropractic care. On my most recent visit with her, unfortunately now at the hospital, she said to me "the best part of this visit was my Chiropractic adjustment."

I hugged and kissed her, and said, "I'll give you another one soon Grandma." My greatest success has been sharing my philosophies with family, and watching them grow and flourish because of these practices. Look long and hard at what turns your crank. Find out what keeps you going, what inspires you, what you want to do for others. Remember, you can't give what you don't have. Start at the beginning, start with YOU.

C.A.N.I.

The powerful play of life goes on and you may contribute a verse – which verse will that be?
~ *Robin Williams, Dead Poet's Society*

Anthony Robbins, one of my mentors, developed the acronym "CANI" more than a decade ago. It stands for Constant And Never-ending Improvement. It is Tony's belief that if all you did were improve one tiny aspect of your life every single day, you would achieve mastery in uncommon time. I would like to share with you some of my 'tiny aspects' that I have incorporated and share regularly with my patients:

- ♦ If you're not getting adjusted regularly, start. Facilitate the 'mind body" connection and be free of nerve interference.
- ♦ It is all about who we "BE" as a person, not what we "HAVE" or "DO."
- ♦ Identify, revisit, and follow your passions.
- ♦ You attract into your life what you think about. Mike Dooley says: "Thoughts become things... choose the good ones."
- ♦ Have goals that are S.M.A.R.T. (specific, measurable, attainable, and realistic, and with a time frame) and aligned with your values, beliefs and passions.
- ♦ Life is about the celebrating the 'moments' along the journey of 'life'.
- ♦ Adopt an attitude of gratitude.
- ♦ Dream BIG!!
- ♦ Allow your spirit to soar (sing, dance, meditate, yoga, breathe).
- ♦ Exercise, it doesn't matter what it is, just that it is.
- ♦ Nutrition: eat as much green, organic and raw foods as possible.
- ♦ Remember, your best quality sleep starts before midnight.
- ♦ Most of all have fun and laugh – everyday.

It's what's inside of us: our passions, our certainty, and our enthusiasm that feeds our soul. I have such gratitude for the wonderful people and successes in my life. Emerson sums it up beautifully for me:

> To share often and much... to know even one life has breathed easier because you have lived; this is to have succeeded.
> ~ *Ralph Waldo Emerson*

Have an extraordinary and passionate life!

- **With passion, persistence and discipline anything is possible.**
- **Transformation is an inside job – the "Be-Do-Have."**
- **Bear witness to miracles and marvels.**
- **Find joy and fulfillment.**
- **C.A.N.I.**

17

Now Is The Time
Dr. Denise Perron

> Life is not easy for any of us. But what of that? We must
> have perseverance and above all confidence in ourselves.
> We must believe that we are gifted for something and that
> this thing must be attained.
> ~ Marie Curie

Yes, what of that? Life would be quite dull if it was so *easy-
breezy*, if there were no hurdles or obstacles to endure. The
power of perseverance to get through and over an obstacle
or quandary is what makes achievement so rewarding. Is
that not common knowledge by now? The secret here is: you
really do have to believe it and live it for it to become a truth
in your life. This can be applied to our personal, spiritual and
physical lives.

Now Is The Time For
Individual Consciousness Over Our Health

We live during a time in our planet's history where the
health of our population must be placed at the apex of our
priority list. The world has grown too many poisons for us to
ignore them any longer. Being a Chiropractic healer, living
everyday with the Chiropractic Principles has given me the
strength and ability to help so many people – including my
family, loved ones, and of course, myself.

The truth is, we all have this gift within us: to heal ourselves through vitalism and balance in our lives. It's time all of us take conscientiousness of our imminent health. This consciousness must stem from the belief and confidence in ourselves to possess this power to embrace it and to use it as an influence over our health. And on a more basic level, to act in a way we all already know is right. We now know so much about the perfect balance between good nutrition, exercise, relaxation, elimination of toxic substances/influences and mental stimulation. Is it not time to fully benefit from all this education and knowledge?

Now that we have the tools, we can finally become a major influence on our health and subsequently, health and purity in our bodies is needed to operate a balanced vessel, a successful life, and a happy existence. The real challenge and fun is getting us from the knowing to the doing, to the being in the actions of better health.

Take Control And You Will
Benefit So Much More From Chiropractic

Chiropractic helps maintain health, and I believe the future of the caregivers lies in a more supportive role, specifically in reinforcing good lifestyles. There are no miracles; a healthy lifestyle with Chiropractic care can lead and become the way to optimal health. An unhealthy lifestyle cannot all of a sudden be resolved by Chiropractic alone. Chiropractic is part of the solution and a major contributor; however, health is multifaceted and there are multiple aspects that contribute to optimal health.

This truth is what I always emphasize to my patients. Every day activities and everyday life affect your health; you have to make that conscious decision and have to want to help yourself first before relying on anyone or anything. I stress two points. First, maintaining a positive attitude is everything; stress and negativity is the reason for many dysfunctions of the body. Second, although you visit a Chiropractor to be adjusted, it is up to you to maintain a healthy lifestyle. For example, your teeth will only be in good condition when you brush every day. A dentist visit is for maintenance, but brushing everyday is what will bring you the most permanent results. It is quite logical. Taking care of your lifestyle is making sure you will benefit fully from the help of Chiropractic care. In essence, all my patients have come to know this fundamental approach to their pursuit of health.

Taking A Moment To Reboot...

Many times in my life, I have had to *reboot*. Reboot to me is the term I use to refresh my values, and to take a real close look at my lifestyle at that specific point in my life. It is human nature to slip and accepting this is a lesson in itself.

A few years ago, at my office, I experience an enlightening event. My days at the clinic are procedural and planned to the minute. I realized I was going through motions and was achieving great things, yet had omitted the most important: the component of *being* and *valuing*. I decided to expand out of my comfort zone, what I call self-induced CHANGE. Change brings on growth and without it, we stagnate. I changed our office around. I took on new challenges professionally, where I would have to learn and do things I had never done before. And more importantly, I sat down with family and staff members, and humbly created a plan for growth and improvement. Rebooting was really like pressing reset on an electronic devise. It served as a chance to start a new chapter and create opportunities for myself professionally and personally. Also, when I train myself to self-inflict CHANGE, I can be more ready for CHANGE in circumstances I do not control directly.

Unexpected and impromptu situations are part of all of our lives and the difficulty is to put yourself in a mental state where you know, it will be okay and that faced with unforeseeable circumstances, you will overcome, learn and forgive. Only then can you truly reboot.

I Am A Woman, Mother, Wife And Healer

We as women are natural nurturers and healers... I am a mother, a wife, but also a healer. As a woman Chiropractor, there is so much opportunity if you choose to see it. This century has been a real growth spurt for women in most professions, including Chiropractic, and now I feel like there is even more we can build upon. In difficult times, I have found great inspiration in looking at my women predecessors and how much they fought to practice and build careers in Chiropractic, despite political struggles and discrimination. They kept true to their beliefs.

As a Chiropractic student, I had my own obstacles to face. I was a single mom, with debt and an overwhelming schedule and curriculum. My storm slowly past, but only thanks to the inspiration of many women around me and past, who lived through their own stormy hardships. One of my last exams was three days after I gave birth. In the midst of the stress of my examination, my physical pain, and the breast-feeding break outside in the hall, I found relief in a feeling of nurturing. I thought to myself, "We as women are natural nurturers and healers... I am a mother, a wife, but also a healer." The desire and strength to nurture my newborn baby is the same power and strength behind becoming a great Chiropractor and a great healer. I thought, "If only I could apply this strength to Chiropractic, I will succeed. There is only one way to go and that is up!"

The true calling of letting go and understanding the innate power of healing comes when innate runs through your veins and guides you to where you are meant to be. Listening to my innate within, three days after giving birth, I wrote my exams and passed with flying colors. I still don't really know how I did it, only that my sense of purpose was greater than my immediate fears. I wanted to be a Chiropractor, and offered myself to the Universe to be exactly that.

Understanding this is simply an example of how our minds and neurology well adjusted can lead us to where we need to be. We need to show up and we need to be open and ready for the adventures ahead, to trust the Universe will guide us to our rightful place. From that moment on, there has never been a doubt in my mind, wherever I have been in my life was the perfect place to be in order to prepare myself for the next adventure in my life. Same thing applies to the concept of healing with my patients. When I adjust them, I am sure the adjustment leads them to reaching their health potential, and I believe the adjustment is one stone on their path towards health and vitality in their lives. When we (and patients) choose to live our lives, adjusted and committed to maximum health, the journey becomes enjoyable as the realization that health or life is not a destination, but a journey.

I was recently called on a new adventure where, through Chiropractic, I had the idea of creating a shaper with the concept of resistance; it is called *Shatobu*. With the same energy and philosophy, I embrace this new venture, allowing change to make me uncomfortable, learning new skills in business – such as the process of patenting, and unexpected legal issues. It has been such a learning experience, at times quite challenging, but oh-so rewarding! Getting through this part of my life is important for me to share with others. It is proof to me that we as women, and really as humans have the strength to overcome obstacles that seem almost *Everest-like* if we train our minds to follow the true path of what we really believe in. I realize this concept is much like our Chiropractic and healing process: from discomfort, into action to alleviate the discomfort. Find the source of the pain and adjust the mind, body and spirit so the intent and values are expressed.

My values are the same with my new adventure as they are with Chiropractic: the desire to serve more people.

Through *SHATOBU* I can give women the edge in their exercise programs. Through Chiropractic, I help my patients achieve their maximum health potential.

I know so many women in the world – in Chiropractic and out of Chiropractic – that are living these Principles and are mentors for me. Find them in your life, reach out to them, and model them. Greatness comes from greatness and it is your birthright. Enjoy your journey, show the best of your abilities and be aligned, adjusted with your values. Be the flame you want to be and be sure to express your potential everyday. What is most important is to *show up* everyday, as best you can! *You can and will make a difference!*

> I am only one, but still I am one; I cannot do everything but still can do something. And because I cannot do everything, I will not refuse to do the something I can do.
> ~ *Helen Keller*

- **Now is the time for individual consciousness over our health.**
- **Truth is, we all have this gift within us.**
- **Take control and you will benefit so much more from Chiropractic.**
- **We as women are natural nurturers and healers.**

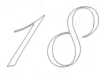

Tale Of Trust
Dr. Dena Churchill

ChiropracTic. The tic, the tock, the timeless clock. My tic in Chiropractic is the timelessness of the message – a message that states there is an innate wisdom in the Universe that heals the body and that Chiropractic removes the interference to allow this Intelligence. After 15 years in practice and thousands of patients, I am now beginning to understand the full ramifications of this message: to be confident enough to share what I know; to stay humble to learn what I do not know; and to have the courage to listen first with my heart.

Innate wisdom... what is this? This is the spirit of healing. Spirit is Universal Intelligence, an intangible energy that encompasses us all, creates night and day and the seasons; allows a fetus to develop (even when it does not yet have a brain); and supports life of a cell without a nucleus. We can't see this energy, but by deduction in science, now know it exists. Everything is guided by this Universal power.

The nervous system, being one of the first tissues to develop, allows for the growth and differentiation of all other systems. It innervates all the cells, tissues and organs in the body and is the carrier of this wisdom from the brain to the body, from embryo to elderly. As Chiropractors we have the privilege to unleash this power through our nervous system optimizing our human potential.

We all know the symptom benefits of Chiropractic care. But what I may not be able to quantify in a patient file and report is the most life changing aspect. The impact on health potential, social interactions, relationships, minds and emotions is the miracle woven into the healing transformation that holds the vitality of life.

Women hold a unique container for this wisdom in our nurturing, mothering intuitive existence. Caring, trusting and knowing places women at the forefront of many healthcare decisions. Men and women learn from each other and together create life, but women supporting women births and nurses the next generation.

Confucius states that wisdom is the love of learning through "reflection (the noblest), imitation (the easiest), and experience (the bitterest)." Through sharing my humble experiences and reflections, my wish for you, the reader, is that it may provide you with a wink of wisdom into the power of Chiropractic.

Tale OF Trust

This first story is about twenty-six-year-old Jamie, who is encouraged by her mother to have a Chiropractic spinal screening exam. Her mother has had success with Chiropractic and wants the same for her daughter. There are no symptoms in the history, no reported traumas, surgeries and the daughter reports that she is just here to appease his mother. Upon examination Jamie has one of the most subluxated cervical spines I have palpated in four months!

"Jamie, are you sure there has been no physical trauma such as falls, motor vehicle accidents, birth trauma, sports injuries?"

"No, nothing," is the reply.

I am so disillusioned by the discrepancy in what I am palpating and what she is reporting that I go to the waiting room to ask her mother the same questions. "Mrs. S, are you sure Jamie has had no trauma?"

She at first doesn't volunteer any memory.

Jokingly I say, "It feels as though she was dropped on her head as a baby."

After a few minutes, her reply is shocking. "Actually, when she was three months old her brother dropped a 50 lbs mirror on her head. She went unconscious, but by the time we reached the Emergency ward, everything was fine."

"Fine" means they checked her vitals, she was crying and breathing, so they sent her home. There was no spinal exam performed.

I begin to explain to Jamie the importance of treatment, and she decides to trust in her mother's experience and me, and "give this Chiropractic thing a try." After six to eight treatments, one day Jamie says something to me that brings tears to my eyes and opens my heart as to why I am serving in Chiropractic.

"Dr. Churchill, remember on the first visit you asked me if I had headaches and I said I didn't? Well, I think I have had a headache my whole life and didn't know it. My grades are improving; I have more energy and I am sleeping better since the treatments." This story sparks inspiration to tell the optimal living story to all I meet, not waiting twenty-six years for the first spinal check.

Moral of this story: Trust in your palpation and intuition, keep questioning until you find an answer that is congruent and be inspired to share the optimal living story from birth.

> Loving service is offering information and hope, wisdom is honoring informed choice.
> ~ *Dr. Dena Churchill*

A patient, Allison, an audiologist, reports that the tube placed in her daughter's left ear is not draining. I encourage her to bring in her daughter, Erin for a spinal check.

"Can Chiropractic help with ear infections?" she asks.

I reply, "If there is irritation of the cervical nerve roots it may be impeding drainage from the middle ear, it is definitely worth an assessment. A healthy nervous system nourishes a healthy body."

Editorial note: There are many concepts behind why we are seeing remarkable results in these cases. The concepts range from impacting neurology affecting lymphatic drainage, immune modulation, muscle tone changes, to name a few.

Below is a copy of the mother's account of what happens next.

Dear Dr. Dena,

As you know Erin has suffered from ear infections since she was five months old. She has been on antibiotics several times and had ventilation tubes inserted at 14 months of age. The tubes have helped the right ear but the left ear still gets infected every few months. The tube in the left ear gets blocked with debris and an ear infection usually results. The left tube has now been blocked for more than six months. Fluid has built-up in the middle ear and hasn't been able to drain due to the malfunctioning ventilation tube and the malfunctioning eustachian tube.

As an audiologist I'm able to check her tympanograms on a regular basis. Tympanomgrams measure eardrum mobility and middle ear pressure. Normal mobility is between 0.3 and 1.8mL. Erin's left tympanogram has consistently measured 0.1mL suggesting fluid build-up in the middle ear. This measurement has not changed since I started measuring it at five months of age.

After discussing Chiropractic treatment for ear infections with you, we decided to give it a try since we've been battling these ear infections for two years now. She had her first treatment last week.

The following day I measured her tymp. (tympanic membrane motion] and it was 0.2mL. This is a very slight improvement, but an improvement none-the-less! She had her second treatment this week, and again I measured her tymp. the following day. It measured 0.6mL! This is well within normal and suggests that the fluid is no longer sitting in her middle ear.

Parents of children with chronic ear infections don't get a lot of sleep. Erin has not consistently slept through the night since the day she was born; therefore Alex and I have not either. It has now been 10 days since her first treatment and she has since slept 12 hours a night every night, except one. We are absolutely thrilled and want to thank you so much!

Allison

Erin covers her ears now for a different reason, as her world is suddenly *too loud*. Erin and Allison are now both regular wellness patients.

This parent note and inquisition as to why there is very little communication with the medical profession inspired me to pursue this as a project. Allison is a practitioner measuring auditory function of hundreds of children per month and didn't know the benefits of Chiropractic treatment for Otitis Media. On a mission to share this story in an Otolaryngology Journal, I began communication with the research department library at the Canadian Chiropractic College, the IWK Children's Hospital and the provinces local Nova Scotia Hearing and Speech Departments; but there was resistance in this process and destiny was dictating a different direction. I voiced my concerns to a pediatric Chiropractor that gave me the following heartfelt advice:

Our purpose in Chiropractic should be focused on removing interference to the full expression of the optimal State of Wellbeing. That is not the treatment of symptoms, conditions, or diseases. Yes, people do almost invariably get symptomatically better as a result of receiving specific Chiropractic adjustments. But, I do make it clear to each new person in our practice that this is the result of their whole-being better performing the functions of life (self-healing & self-regulating), and not because we have some secret treatment that no one else knows about. I don't think our obligation is to educate one or any number of ENTs, but to educate the people about what we really do in affecting their 'State of Wellbeing.'

~ *Dr. Eddy Cohen*

Moral of the story: Never promise results, but offer a possibility for health. Loving service is an offering. Wisdom is honouring those that inspire you but respecting that some may not be ready for your message.

Ask For A Healing Invitation
And Allow The Patient A Voice

Nine-year-old twins present to the office with behavioral concerns diagnosed as ADHD. Years of school suspensions, meeting with social workers and psychologists, taking medication, 'out-of control' behaviors and the parents came to me as a last resort.

Matthew is vibrating into my office on the first visit. He is not able to maintain eye contact and before I can answer one question he is onto the next. His skin is so sensitive he couldn't tolerate a handshake, so I greet him by shaking his leg. We get through the history and exam, and I discuss with Matthew my findings, the benefits of Chiropractic and the treatment.

The invitation to healing must be set between the practitioner and the patient, regardless of the age. The consent form covers your legal obligation, but in this sacred healing space you must be invited-in by the patient: talk to the minor; show them the tools you are using; honor wherever they are at that time. Sacred Healing Laws of the Universe require this non-verbal contract of trust and consent.

When I put my hands on Matthew to adjust him for the first time in an hour, he is silent. I continue. He is lying supine as I perform a toggle adjustment on his neck and he remains silent. Mother makes eye contact with me and shrugs her shoulders at my inquiring glance. Once we finish, I sit for a few minutes in the silence; then tell Matthew we are finished and he may slowly sit up when he is ready. He stands up and then has a reaction that neither of us is expecting.

He begins to scream, "Aahhh, I feel straight and I do not want to be straight, I don't like this feeling. I am scared. I want to die! Please, please put me back the way I was." He is holding his head between his hand pacing back and forth the treatment room as his mother is trying to calm him without success, and his father and twin brother come in from the waiting room to see why there is crying and screams.

I gently lower my voice so the tension in the room must meet me to re-connect with Matthew. "Matthew what is it that I can do to help you? What is it you are feeling?"

"Everything is quiet and it is scary and I don't want to be this way; please put me back the way I was."

Trying to find words of comfort I say, "Matthew, Chiropractic is about freeing nervous system irritation and restoring motion, but if you give it a few days without anymore treatment likely it will return to how it was."

He is obviously calmer, understanding I was listening and trying to respect his wishes. I sit next to him on the table and thank him for the opportunity to work with him. I explain that he will no longer be visiting the office, as the service I am offering is not what he seeks. The mother is not understanding the shift in power I am creating with my reverse psychology and is crying and pleading with Matthew to give it a chance. I am firm in pointing out that the decision is Matthew's.

Matthew replies with a phrase that opens my heart and my eyes to the power of Chiropractic, "Doc, this change is scary, but please, I really want to come back here again, could you just make me half straight?"

This boy's nervous system had been vibrating at this frequency for years, but the moment of silence from the Chiropractic adjustment scares him into hysterics. Even through his fear, his words suggest an intuitive knowing of the power in Chiropractic as a healing modality and he wishes to continue at a slower pace.

His mother, father and twin brother, who I thought would be running scared by Matthew's response, all booked-in for new patient visits before they left the office. There is a profound change in Matthew that is felt and respected by everyone in the room.

To be a facilitator in this healing transformation is awe-inspiring.

The moral of this story: There is great power in the Chiropractic adjustment; connect and respect the patient regardless of their age.

Transforming Language

Our words are the connection between our imagined thoughts and our actions of reality. They reflect our thoughts, allow us to communicate with our environment and seed the earth to grow towards our destiny. Thus, transforming our language is the most efficient blueprint to creating health destiny. What you say to the patient and what they say to themselves matters. If a patient says, "I am tight and sore," I repeat it back to them with the result I'd love, "I see you are becoming stronger and more flexible with each treatment." The intention of these words has the power to change beliefs and thoughts and create new realities.

Pain or a spinal subluxation is just a feedback mechanism. It creates imbalance, and through this polarity we create a potential for health. Health is never static. It is this dynamic differential that adds life's color and excitement. Love the subluxations for the opportunity to grow, learn and teach your patients the value in listening to their body. A Chiropractic mentor once said he would never wish the patient to be pain free, for it is often pain or discomfort that changes behavior. Greater body-mind awareness is the power of healing.

The conversation of the mind and body is an emerging field of study. Most understand the mind and emotions creating a physiological response. The *fight or flight* response is a sympathetic nervous system example to which many will relate. You experience fear and your heart begins to race, and your tissues become hypertonic. But in liberating a restriction in the physical body you may also produce emotions.

Dr. Candace Pert's molecules of emotion are neuropeptides that may be released in tissue memory of the physical body and may also liberate an emotion. Awareness of these phenomena is an example of quantum healing in Chiropractic. When both the patient and the doctor hold this holistic perspective, understanding the purpose of pain as just a feedback mechanism to a body and mind, then each day is a journey of adventure.

The book you are reading reminds me of the Anita Diamant book entitled, *The Red Tent*. It is grounded in the ancient knowledge that when women gather in the spirit of sharing, joy and healing, wondrous things happen.

The following is a note, I wrote April 23, 2010 for the women gathered at *The Red Tent* Event.

Radiance:
The power is within you. You are the doctor of your ills, the designer of your destiny, the reflector of the radiance that flows through you. It is our fears that create obstacles and illusions that serve to disempower. Our own shadow holds us captive. To see the wall, understand why there are different perspectives, and transcend all perceptions is the key to finding love and grace, gaining an infinite wisdom to create.

May this book of Women in ChipropracTic offer you love and wisdom wherever you are in your journey, giving you the confidence to share what you know, the reminder to stay humble to learn what you do not know, and the courage to first listen with your heart.

- **Appreciate the power of the adjustment.**
- **Trust your skills and blend with intuition.**
- **Women bring nurturing and mothering instincts.**
- **You offer hope and possibility.**
- **Honor informed choice.**
- **Connect and respect the patient regardless of age.**

Honoring The Voice Within
Dr. Jeanne Ohm

Growing up on Long Island in the Sixties and Seventies meant growing up fast and furiously during an uncertain and tumultuous time. All of society was being challenged and new concepts and philosophies were being introduced and experimented with. It was a time of recognized repression, consequent rebellion, and demonstrative expectation for change. It has been said that out of chaos comes creation. During those challenging days, like many, I found myself delving within and asking deep, soul-searching questions.

And so even at a young age, I began to ask the questions of the ages. "Who are we?" "Why are we here?" "What is here?" "Is this our only life?" "What is our Source?" "Where is our Source?" "What is our relationship?" "Are we in the right relation?" I spent hours pouring over these questions and the myriad of possible answers with my best friend, soon to be husband, Tom. We delved into world religions, texts, philosophies and teachings. We discussed, pondered, argued and contemplated. And we came away convinced of a higher Universal Intelligence pervading and expressing itself in earth.

Practical application came slower and the dots began to connect when I was first introduced to Chiropractic. At nineteen years of age, I jumped off a cliff while hang-gliding and dove to the ground faster than I could have imagined. Fracturing two vertebrae in my spine was one of the biggest pattern interrupts in my life... my enthusiasm, trust and free flowing expression was suddenly halted with the sudden physical injury I sustained. After a full year of medical intervention – still plagued with daily pain – someone suggested I go to a Chiropractor.

Hearing The Chiropractic Story

Knowing little about Chiropractic and basing this decision on a friend's referral, we walked into an office seeking care and met a man who embraced the philosophy, science and art of Chiropractic. Before he even allowed us to begin care, he insisted on us coming to a class on Chiropractic Philosophy. There Tom and I sat learning the Principles of Chiropractic...starting with the major premise, *"There is a Universal intelligence in all matter, continuously giving to it all its properties and actions, thus maintaining it in existence, and giving this intelligence its expression."* He continued with another Principle: *"A living thing has the intelligence of the Universe inborn within it, referred to as its innate intelligence."*

Tom and I sat higher in our seats... this was quite the interesting evening. We went in for treatment for our bad backs and this man was discussing Universal Principles and vitalistic philosophy? Where was the connection...was there a connection?

The Chiropractor continued, "The function of the body's Innate Intelligence is to adapt Universal forces and matter for use in the body, so that all parts of the body will have coordinated action for mutual benefit, however there can be interference with the transmission of innate forces. This interference with the transmission of innate forces causes discoordination, or *dis*-ease.

And then he made the powerful connection of the expression of this Intelligence in our bodies. "Some of the forces the body's Innate Intelligence creates operate through or over

the nerve system in animal bodies. Interference with transmission in the body is often directly or indirectly due to
subluxations in the spinal column." Several months later, our
fires lit and purpose confirmed; we decided to become Chiropractors.

Vitalism In Physical Health

For Tom, this philosophy of trusting the Intelligence of the
body was supported by his family's way of life. They rarely
went to doctors, they expected the body to heal on its own
and any procedure short of major surgery was cared for with
home remedies. I can recall walking into the kitchen and one
of the brothers was being bandaged by another. I can recall
his father explain that when he had a fever, he would wrap
himself up in numerous layers of clothes and blankets to
burn the fever out. There was no attempt to lower the tem-
perature and make the body's job harder. Rather he had a
trust in the body's ability to innately know what was best.
With humility, he followed that natural course, supporting its
inherent wisdom.

For me, this philosophy had not been applied to the body
in my childhood. I had three major surgeries by the time I
was six. When my sister was born, my father insisted that all
visitors wear a 'germ' mask. We sneezed and we went to the
doctor. Perhaps it was because my father was a health insurance salesman. At any rate, I grew up in a very mechanistic
paradigm of fear.

Having now been introduced to a vitalistic philosophy of
life and having it connected to the physical realm with Chiropractic, Tom and I approached our family values from the
perspective of trust. Easier for him then me... this was the
beginnings of a learning process that would be tested time
and time again.

When pregnant with our first child, we decided to have a home birth. My previous experiences with hospitals had not reinforced trust in the system; they had rather introduced a deep fear and aversion to hospitals and technology. I can remember announcing to his parents, my mother, her husband, my father and his wife that we would be having an unattended home birth. The conversation went from excitement over our pregnancy to disdain, criticism and chaos.

Tom and I listened to the uproar and when they had all finished bursting their reproaches, I announced, "If we are going to argue for the duration of this pregnancy every time we see each other, then I think it will be best for us to discontinue communication until after the baby is born."

I knew the importance of surrounding myself with support and encouragement in pregnancy in preparation for a safer, easier birth and my maternal intuition was surfacing in protection. My mother could not bear the thought of not talking for nine months, and so the remainder of our pregnancy was somewhat peaceful.

When Justin was born, my father's wife, a head nurse in a NY hospital, insisted on coming down to check on him herself. Much to her surprise, our son and I were healthy and safe.

When we conceived our second child, my father asked, "So are you over this *homebirth fad* yet? You will be having this one in a hospital, right?" Shifting paradigms and core beliefs are hard for parents to accept.

So we had our six children at home, slept with them, consistently carried them and breastfed them for over a year even before the coined terms: *unattended homebirth, co-sleeping, baby wearing* and *exclusive breastfeeding*. We did this because we were following our innate guidance directing us from our core beliefs. When parents ask me how did we know to birth naturally, avoid vaccinations, allow fevers and infections to run their course, filter our water, and so forth, I explain it all comes down to identifying core beliefs and holding all decisions up to them.

Essentially, there are two perspectives about healing. One is mechanistic – it defines life as a random series of events, devoid of an organized and intelligent purpose. Sickness is to be treated, symptoms are to be eliminated, and the body needs expert outside opinions based on limited knowledge to help it heal. The other is vitalistic. It recognizes, respects, and trusts in the Intelligence of life and the interconnectedness of this wisdom among all life. Processes of the body are to be trusted, and supported where an underlying confidence for healing and proper function is emphasized.

Hippocrates, the father of medicine, summed up the heart of this perspective well:

> Humans are created to be healthy as long as they are whole: body, mind, spirit. People are characterized by self-healing properties that come from within—an innate healing force. Perfect health and harmony is the normal state for all life.

It is imperative that we define our core values and consciously make our life and health choices from the perspective which resonates best with those values. It is also imperative for us to choose practitioners who base their choices on the same foundation.

As we are learning to discern between vitalism and mechanism, it is important to become familiar with the tenets of vitalistic care:

- ◆ Vitalism recognizes the existence of an Intelligence organizing and coordinating all function.
- ◆ Vitalistic care respects and trusts this wisdom.
- ◆ Vitalistic care focuses on naturally supporting and enhancing overall normal body function rather than the chemical alteration of symptoms with drugs.

- ◆ Vitalistic approaches recognize that the body has the inherent wisdom to function normally and that physical, emotional and chemical stressors may overload the body's ability to do so. The goal is to remove these stressors, allowing the body to return to balanced function.
- ◆ Symptoms are recognized as body alerts that serve to reveal stress overload. From the vitalistic perspective, it is not important to label the condition, and it is considered counterproductive to silence these symptoms with drugs.
- ◆ Vitalistic care is not the diagnosis or treatment of conditions and diseases. Rather, it is a process of identifying and eliminating the cause of the body's overload. Only when the overload has been eliminated can a person experience wellness.
- ◆ Finally, the vitalistic, proactive approach is encouraged before symptoms even appear. In the case of Chiropractic Wellness Care, spinal checks are encouraged to enhance nervous system function and overall health, with or without symptoms.

Our kids were generally very healthy and always well. Yes, we attributed it to the "Chiropractic family wellness lifestyle" of natural birth, good foods, lots of movement, positive emotional environment, and regular adjustments. And we also attributed it to our broader definition of health that included wellness. When they had fevers, infections, and colds we considered these to be normal body functions and adaptations to the situation at hand, not illness to be diagnosed, treated and ultimately suppressed. I can count on one hand how many times we brought all six kids to a medical doctor. At that time, there were essentially no medical doctors who practiced from a vitalistic perspective. We did not know about homeopathy or naturopathy. We dealt with injuries and 'illnesses' with care and natural, non-suppressive home remedies. We checked their spines to eliminate any interference to their nervous system. We watched, waited and trusted, supporting the body in its inherent ability to heal and be well.

Shifting to this paradigm is sometimes challenging, especially since the majority of the healthcare industry, news media, laws, regulations and yes, even our own families do not support this perspective. It is hard to go against the grain, and we are often met with resistance, opposition, and outright criticism, laced with fear and even intimidation. That paralyzing emotion – *fear* – then becomes the motivating factor for decisions. But fear is too volatile an emotion from which to make any good choices. I am reminded of the quote from Bertrand Russell:

> Collective fear stimulates herd instinct, and tends to produce ferocity toward those who are not regarded as members of the herd.

This has been the basis for allopathic care in the Western world.

In thirty years of making life and health choices for our family, my husband and I have heard all of the arguments used to challenge our vitalistic core beliefs. When we started having our family, there was little to no peer-reviewed evidenced based research on natural birthing, co-sleeping, long-term breastfeeding, vaccination risks, and the refusal of drugs for symptomatic relief. We were labeled irresponsible at best. We were told our beliefs had no scientific validation. Since then, however, research has shown otherwise.

Even more importantly, to us, both then and now, credibility does not come from a limited mechanistic science devoid of any recognition of vitalism. A new emerging science is offering validation for the essential Principles of Vitalism. It is less known and only sparsely integrated into the healing arts. Bruce Lipton, PhD, author of Biology of Belief terms it "the new edged science." It is a science now substantiating the philosophy we embrace. Max Planck, Nobel Prize–winning physicist and the father of quantum theory, acknowledged this new science well in a 1944 speech:

> All matter originates and exists only by virtue of a force....
> We must assume behind this force the existence of a conscious and intelligent mind. This mind is the matrix of all matter.

Since then, and now in the 21st century, the relationship between this emerging science and health is becoming more sought out and integrated. Although promoted over 100 years ago by the founder of Chiropractic, D.D. Palmer, the recognition and practice of healthcare from an inherent trust of our amalgamation with a greater intelligence is finally being embraced. Deepak Chopra, MD, sums up this principle well:

> There is an inner intelligence in your body, and that inner intelligence is consciousness. It's the ultimate in supreme genius, which mirrors the wisdom of the Universe.

Vitalism in Parenting Values

As parents, Tom and I took vitalism one step further, beyond our physical well-being and into the realm of our parenting lifestyle. There's a *Moody Blues* album from the late Sixties entitled *To Our Children's Children's Children*. My husband Tom and I used to listen to it frequently. Their songs reflected hope and vision for a new generation of social and spiritual change. When we were still kids, we would spend hours talking about our vitalistic philosophy of life. One day in high school, we skipped classes and spent the entire day discussing "how kids should be raised." Being kids ourselves, and still intimate with that perspective, we outlined some essentials.

First and foremost, we agreed kids are born inherently good and that they are seeking to express their own, innate potential. Allowing this to manifest requires a sense of trust in a greater good, and a respect for a higher intelligence connecting and overseeing the expression of all life, kids included. We recognized kids have their own soul's purpose to fulfill, and they are here to teach parents as much as parents are here to teach them. In other words, the relationship is multidimensional, and the parameters of 'right and wrong' are not a polarized black-and-white set of rules, but rather many hues of color, depending on each moment in time.

That lead us to our next conclusion: The *spirit* of the law, not the letter of the law, should be the determining factor in making rules and enforcing boundaries. Each situation brings its own set of circumstances, and decisions should be adapted to the situation at hand. Parenting requires the ability to shift perspectives, adapt ideas and yes, embrace continued growth and change.

When Tom and I were introduced to Chiropractic at nineteen years of age, specific spinal adjustments facilitated my healing from a serious injury and also eliminated lifelong symptoms of headaches, asthma and intense allergies. It was, however, the philosophy of Chiropractic that inspired us to become Chiropractors. Here we saw a perspective that recognizes an Innate Intelligence in all living things, a wisdom overseeing and coordinating function on all levels: physical, emotional and spiritual. From the traditional teachings of Chiropractic, we learned trust and respect for the natural process of life in all situations. We were fortunate to be introduced to the essence of the Chiropractic Philosophy as being far beyond "healthcare." It's a way of life.

After Tom and I married we had six wonderful, expressive and happy kids. We offered an environment of love and security by honoring the child and choosing our birthing, feeding and bonding styles to validate our respect for them as well. We, like many Chiropractic families, chose these approaches because they respected the evolution and expressions of a child's own innate potential and his or her importance as an individual expressive soul. These ideals are consistent with our philosophy of life, as well as the Chiropractic Philosophy of honoring our innate wisdom.

As our children grew older, we continued this trust and respect by allowing them to co-create the parameters of our home 'boundaries.' Communication between parents and children in our house is safe, open and very dynamic, with everyone's input expressed, heard and considered. Even if choices are made that we do not wholeheartedly agree with, we often allow them so we can all learn and grow together. And so we do.

We continue to realize children are born with an inherent connection to their source – a deep, inherent wisdom untainted by worldly ways. Allowing them to live and express this wisdom helps us stay connected to our source as well.

Vitalism In Practice

Not too long ago, a father in our practice said to me, "I'm afraid *not* to vaccinate, and I'm just as afraid *to* vaccinate." My response was not to address the list of pros and cons on either side of the vaccination issue. Apparently he had already done that. Had he not, I would have first suggested resources for him to explore. Since he had apparently already weighed the option and come away with fear and indecision, my response was instead to have him take two steps back, and understand that any choice made from fear is made from a skewed perspective and would be unproductive and disconnected from source. Rather than building on this unstable foundation created by fear, it was more important for him to define his core values in life – those essential values from which all of his life decisions could be made. Once defined, he would be making a decision from a place of certainty and trust.

In practice, it is imperative to offer information for parents to become informed. They need to read the facts, the research, the stories, and express concerns from either side.

Ultimately, however to make a decision they can truly stand behind, they need to go deeper than 'informed choice,' they need to reach a level of 'conscious choice.'

Chiropractors have been known to be excellent educators. It was Chiropractors who first brought significant attention to nutrition, exercise, and positive attitude long before the mass mind of health care caught on. We have been leaders in sparking social awareness about vaccinations, medications, and technological births all by introducing Chiropractic Vitalistic Principles that make sense. But teaching about the dangers of routine medical practices and showing the logical approach of how the body functions, adapts, heals and regenerates only reaches the mental realm of the person. Referring to the root of the word education, it means to "draw forth." Ideas are not drawn forth; they are shared, pondered, learned. To draw forth, means to go to a deeper state of being than the mental state. It means to reach into a place of belief, commitment, and core value.

As for the father in my practice choosing to vaccinate or not, I don't know for sure what he chose. As a practitioner, I must free up the parents to make their own "conscious choices." What I can and did do was direct him to the importance of connecting with his wife, going within, and embracing their highest knowing. This is our greatest service as educators to all parents who are making life and health choices for their families. First, they need to gather the information available in regard to the decision at hand. Then, they need to move out of the realm of mind, put all of it aside and recognize the essence of their conscious-selves' beliefs. Once they have identified these life Principles, they are ready to weigh their choices from this place of knowing. Choosing from a state of trust and conviction consistent with these essential values become the connection to our inner strength. From this place of certainty, we will always choose correctly.

Connection To The Knowing

For centuries, women's intuition was respected as a vital contribution to the health and well-being of their families. Personal experience through pregnancy and birth lead us to trust in the natural processes of the body's function. Our natural ability to bond with our children gave us great insight into the physical and emotional needs of our families. Women's ability to seek guidance from that quiet place within was honored in those cultures.

In recent years, technology has seemingly replaced women's input in family health decisions. It is not so much the voice of intuition has stopped talking to us, but more accurate to say its validity is being disregarded by our high-tech society. We have been lead from trusting the natural process and hearing its internal messages to looking outside ourselves for support and guidance.

It is time for us to return our attention inward and learn to trust the voice of intuition trying to guide us every day of our lives. I am sure you know what I mean by that voice. Call it "women's intuition," or the "gut feeling" or the "wisdom within." We're all familiar with the terms, but most importantly we've all heard this voice. We've also experienced "going with it" in our lives when it really mattered and that by listening to the voice, things worked out just right. Sometimes it speaks to us on simple and small matters and other times on life threatening matters.

Over the years, many women have shared their stories with us. One friend told us how she was coming up to an intersection in her car. Although the light was green, her gut feeling told her to stop. At the risk of being sworn at by the driver behind her, she stopped at the green light anyway. Just as she did, another car came plowing through the intersection barely missing her. Listening to the voice and its seemingly irrelevant message saved her life!

How many of your own experiences can you recall? How about the times you just knew someone in your family needed you, and you listened to the voice and you found out they did. One man recently shared an experience where a woman he was working with suddenly got up and said, "I've got to call home right now."

When she did, it turned out her husband had been trying to get in touch with her because her child was very ill. The certainty of her knowing and her ability to act on it made a tremendous impression on this man.

He commented to me, "There must be something that happens with you women in pregnancy or birth to keep you so connected with your families."

Yes, this is very true. We have a deep connection with our inner wisdom and therefore our family's well-being. All we have to do is listen and follow its guidance. You see, the more we trust this voice and carry out its wisdom, the stronger and more often it communicates with us.

One woman recently told us how she was supposed to undergo a recommended medical procedure and had procrastinated for months because her gut said no. Because of the pain she had been enduring, she finally gave in to the doctor's recommendation and scheduled an appointment to have it done.

As she sat in the office, she became more and more uneasy. All through her life she had listened to this voice. It's infallible knowing and her trust in that knowing had always worked out for her. As she explained her fears and apprehensions to the doctor, he became increasingly impatient. He finally threatened her that if she were to refuse the procedure at this time, he would discontinue care in the future. With a tremendous amount of strength, she trusted her inner knowing and refused the procedure.

After the doctor stormed out of the room, the two attending nurses gave her the biggest hug and congratulated her decision. Obviously, these two women were familiar with trusting the voice of intuition as well.

Too often we hear stories how mothers just knew something about their child or themselves and were persuaded to believe otherwise. Pressure and intimidation outside of their inner knowing persuaded them to ignore their guidance. The price they paid for being talked out of trusting their intuition often had lifelong consequences.

Birth is one of the most profound examples of how we have allowed the mystique of technology to overcome practical intuition. Before our high tech involvement, women gave birth for centuries without outside interference. Women trusted their intuition and respected their bodies' inherent ability to function as it has been created to. Today, that trust is being squelched and dismissed by many practitioners. What is so special about Chiropractic is that its basic premise includes regaining trust and assurance in the body's Innate Intelligence. Doctors of Chiropractic guide their patients to depend on this inner wisdom. They encourage them to allow the body's Innate healing capacity to express as it is created to, once the nerve system stress has been reduced. Not only do they reconnect their patients with this inner Intelligence through the physical adjustment, they also support parent's need to listen to and follow their own inner wisdom when making health choices for their families. In Chiropractic there is a deep respect for an Intelligence greater than man's finite, educated knowledge.

Honoring The Voice

One of my favorite stories exemplifying listening to this voice comes from the developer of Chiropractic, B.J. Palmer. In his book, *The Bigness Of The Fellow Within* he has this story entitled, "That Something." Written by W.W. Woodbridge, this story reflects a time in the author's life before he "awakened," as he terms it. It was a rough time, filled with strife and discord. He was homeless, poverty stricken, hungry and destitute. When trying to beg for help from a stranger on the street, the stranger replied:

"No," he answered, a note of pity in his voice. "I cannot help you. No man can."

"But you could feed me," I said, with some petulance in my voice.

"It is not food you need!"

"What then?" I asked.

"That Something," was his reply.

The story continues with the author's experience of falling asleep, having a dream and hearing a voice. He questioned the voice:

"Who are you?" I asked.

"I am 'That Something'," came the reply.

"But where are you?"

"I am hidden in your soul."

"How – how did you get there?"

"I was born there."

"Why have I not known you were there before?"

"No man knows it," answered the voice, "until he awakes."

"Are you in other men's souls, as well?"

"There is 'That Something' in every man's soul, which can move the mountains or dry the seas."

"Then you must be Faith!"

"Yes," came the answer, "I am Faith, but I am more – I am that which makes men face the fires of hell, and win."

"Then you must be Confidence, as well."

"Yes, I am more than Confidence – I am that which makes the babbling brooks lift worlds upon their wavelets."

"You are Power," I cried.

"Yes, I am more than Power," answered the voice. "I am that which makes the wretched failure lift up himself and rule the world."

"You are Ambition – I know you now."

"Yes, I am all you say – Faith, Confidence, Power, Ambition, and more. For greater than all is 'That Something.' I am that which every man must find in his soul or else he will be but a clutter of the earth on which he lives."

"But how can man find you?"

"Even as you are finding me now. First you must awaken, then seek, and when you have found you must learn to control . . ."

"Control what?" I asked, confused.

"'That Something' . . . borrow it from your soul and baptize your life with it. Anoint your eyes, that you may see; anoint your ears, that you may hear; anoint your heart, that you may be!"

"But tell me," I cried frantically, for the voice was trailing off to almost nothing, "How can I do this? How? How?"

"This is the secret," came the voice to me as the whisper of a gentle breeze, "These words: *'I will.'*"

The story continues with how the author listened to the voice of That Something and followed its minute-to-minute promptings. By doing so, within one year's time, he not only had a job, but also was approaching the highest level of management in the company. Opportunities and shifts in all areas of his life occurred.

I know throughout my life, when I have listened to this voice, it has led me to creation, success, and fulfillment on all levels of expression.

When it comes to the future of wellness, the shift to vitalism, Moms, I believe it's up to us. Our family wellness begins prior to conception and continues with our choices throughout pregnancy and for birth. Once our children are born, the family wellness lifestyle depends on our continued ability as parents to become informed, discuss this information with our partner and then move from the mind into the sacred space where we can hear the voice. Once heard, we need only say, *"I will."*

Celebrating The Conscious Choice To Vitalism

It is a time of great change. Leaders in science are calling it "The Shift." Leaders in healing are referring to it as the raising of the consciousness. Even politicians are talking about the readiness for our social change and our responsibility as individuals to contribute. Everyone is recognizing that the awareness and participation of each and every one of us is necessary. From a perspective of vitalism, what does that mean?

In times of great change, before the shift occurs, there is usually intense polarization. Fostering the polarization is the use of guilt and fear to maintain the old and fading modes of power. It is important we are aware of these tactics and that we do not fall prey to their influence. This means we must not allow fear and guilt to motivate us to remain motionless, and it also means we must not resort to using these stifling emotions in our zeal to rush the change.

From a vitalistic perspective, this shift is inevitable. It carries its own momentum and will bring a state of balance and ease. Being true to the vitalistic Principle, now is a time for us to trust this process with thoughts and actions consistent with this trust.

Vitalism is described as the recognition that there is a wise and conscious Intelligence within us that reflects the wisdom of the Universe. This wisdom is at the very core of our existence. It is the essence of who we are. In vitalism there is respect of and trust in this wisdom, recognition we are all connected with this wisdom...not just those who agree with us, but everyone. We have a responsibility to ourselves and to others – for the "good of the whole."

Frequently, in times of great change like the one we are living through, we hold on to old learned beliefs with a tight grasp resisting change. When we feel bombarded with these restrictive emotions of fear and guilt, our first response is often to react with like emotions. We then resort to our in-grained patterns of fear and guilt and therefore stifle the potential to hear clear guidance and see empowering options. We must remember that these reactive emotions only serve to stall the momentum for the change we are most desirous of.

The emotion of guilt is strengthened when we are dwelling on the past and the emotion of fear is fed when we are focusing on the future. Both emotions take us from present time consciousness into a pseudo-reality. In this pseudo-reality we sabotage our very creative abilities' potential for change. We must actively shift our focus to present time consciousness.

Equally important to realize is these emotions, fear and guilt, lead to judgment. Judgment is a product of learned thinking, not intuitive guidance. Judgment will also sabotage the potential to creatively shift.

In present time consciousness, we recognize that we always have a choice. Since fear and guilt strengthen our grasp on learned and limiting beliefs, in these states, we resort to automatic behavior and stifle empowering options.

To break this stifling model and to move into present time consciousness, we need only realize that at every moment of our lives, we have the power and permission to choose our perspective.

In his book, the choice, famous author Og Mandino writes:

> Choice! The key is choice. You have options. You need not spend your life wallowing in failure, ignorance, grief, poverty, shame self pity and sickness. But hold on! If this is true, then why have so many among us apparently elected to live in that manner? The answer is obvious. Those who

live in unhappy failure have never exercised their options for a better way of life because they have never been aware that they had any choice!

We can embrace a perspective that fosters respect and trust. We can choose to perceive from a place of gratitude and love. These states of awareness bring us into present time consciousness. They foster respect and trust. They soothe the antagonistic, unfruitful emotions of guilt, fear, and judgment. They create balance and ease. They allow us to connect with our inner wisdom, hear its guidance and give us the strength to say, "I will."

Today, it is up to us to contribute to the shift and rise by finding a state of gratitude and directing our motherly love to our Source, our world, our communities, our families and most of all, That Something within.

- **Symptoms are recognized as body alerts that serve to reveal stress overload.**
- **Trust in a greater good.**
- **Awakening to who we are and what we can be.**
- **There is great value in listening to your inner wisdom.**
- **Honoring the voice, acting on it.**
- **Celebrating vitalism as a conscious choice – living it, applying it.**

Epilogue

This book is not intended to ask you to become a cloned version of any of us or a *"mini-me"* in any way. Rather it is asking you to become the very best version of you!

Let us talk to and support one another. If I may suggest for those who are seasoned, offer to take in a new grad and mentor them. New grads, ask for help and appreciate your elders. They do have a great deal of experience, which counts! If you are able to observe them, listen and look for the nuances. Look for the subtle messages behind the touch and the tone of the words spoken.

Remember to ask for help and then be open to the opportunities that arise. Help others for the sake of being of service, and when you are ready help will come to you in one form or another.

Let go of being a perfectionist. It is an impossible standard to keep. Re-frame to instead strive for excellence. Excellence is a continuously moving bar upwards as we continue to grow and learn each day. It inspires us to always do our very best at any given moment.

It seems to be a paradox in that we go into a profession to help others but we often place ourselves last. We may feel selfish or embarrassed, as though by the nature of our work we feel we should be exempt form the same Laws that govern all life.

While flying in an airplane, we are instructed: "Should the plane pressure drastically change, oxygen masks will fall from the over-head. First, place the oxygen mask on yourselves before assisting others." This can be applied in many ways to our general life. Remember to take "time-out" for yourself. Take care of your needs outside of the practice in order to be full to give when in the practice.

Realize that although every day may not be fulfilling, we can strive to make it so. The interesting contradiction of fulfillment is that you can be just starting practice and excited about what each and every day brings forth and feel quite fulfilled. One can also be in practice for years and unfulfilled. One day you may feel complete and the next you might not. It is part of the journey.

One regret in my education was that I wished I had prior knowledge of the ecology of the planet plus vitalistic, Universal Principles and Laws before entering the academic curriculum. It would have provided a different context in which to learn the subjects such as physiology, neurology, kinesiology, biochemistry and nutrition. My questions would have been centered more on: How does our mind-body interact? What changes neurological plasticity? How do we reflect and adapt to our environment? How does our physiology and function reflect and express that change?

We are so much more than bags of biochemical reactions, chemistry and genes. What controls the expression of genes? What causes a gene to express one way or another? What controls our nervous system? How does change happen? What has to exist for the body to breakdown or heal poorly? Just as we have the gene and germ theories, they are incomplete on their own.

Remember we are unable to separate ourselves from all other forms of life. I would have focused on the magnificent interplay between order and chaos, re-creation and breakdown, structure and function, intangible thoughts or feelings impacting form. It would have put more meaning into why I was learning, and would have changed my orientation from the contemporary Reductionist model to a Vitalistic model. Both are of value.

A common thread through this book is that change is possible and this creates hope – a powerful force.

The contributors' writing was not directed in any way, yet there are common themes and messages underlying. As stated in initial chapters, it is my experience that with all we know, we do not change until we feel it, until it becomes us, until we are moved by something, something has touched us and then it becomes us. We are only too often in our heads and as healers need to be more in our hearts. One of my greatest lessons is to stay in my heart and follow my intuition, which as women we are afforded more often than men.

Data and information without practical experience is philosophy, but when we experience what we teach, we learn, integrate, and become wiser.

There is a communication that cannot be fully explained, but when our hearts open we do the best we can from our training. Our work begins to flow and we become "at ease." Our work is an extension of us and reflects where we are as individuals. When we are expressing our values and *on purpose*, we attract the naturally-right people – staff and patients – into our lives. Days are fulfilled and fun. When we go *off purpose*, our lives and then practice reflect disorganization, breakdown, conflict, challenge and even chaos.

It behooves us to observe ourselves in our work since our outer world is a direct reflection of our inner world. And we have within, the power to change in any direction we choose. We appreciate both the challenges and opportunities and recognize we are co-creators in them.

The Universe provides what we can handle, asks us to tune in, trust the Universe, learn, adapt and grow from the experience versus becoming paralyzed by it. It asks us to trust ourselves and not to judge if a situation changes drastically, or when we lose our way or the situation changes and we lose confidence in our own trust. Each experience builds on a previous, and with our wisdom earlier choices may become different ones later. For many of us, the feeling of providing our trust in someone else feels all wrong. For some, we want to be self-sufficient, independent, stoic and autonomous and have difficulty asking for help for fear of looking weak or stupid or... we are used to people needing us, not the other way around. Yet there are times when we need to ask for supporters in our own lives. They may show up in many forms and this journey is best shared, especially with those who understand the challenges of harmonizing work and home.

We can benefit from finding anchoring points to connect and ground ourselves, allowing us to go beyond what we thought possible. Temper the educated mind with inner wisdom to create harmony. Balance the inner world with the outer, so one becomes an extension of the other and who we are on the inside is expressed on the outside. It does not change for different people, places or events.

Many times, results do not turn out the way we had planned; so we need to continue to trust in the Universe and adapt to what is planned for us. This is not to become subservient to destiny, but as the phrase goes 'when preparation meets any opportunity we have destiny.'

When you follow Innate, does it send you in a direction you feel good about? When you resist it, what happens? Each of us is on a journey of life, but when we connect the dots between each experience, patterns emerge. Messages point us in a direction, we only need to listen and follow.

If there is a burning desire to serve, to do 'good,' the Universe will create opportunities to do so. How often are they dismissed or ignored? Thought of as coincidence? All one has to do is open up to see them. They are always there.

We have more opportunities to change directions, grow, meet new people, move, and explore new horizons than ever before. We can cross study with other professions and bridge the gap in the discussion between thought (formless) and body (form) – on some level, connected via the nervous system.

"Just Do It!"

> Until one is committed, there is hesitancy, the chance to draw back, always ineffectiveness. Concerning all acts of initiative (and creation), there is one elementary truth, the ignorance of which kills countless ideas and splendid plans: that the moment one definitely commits oneself, the providence moves too. A whole stream of events issues from the decision, raising in one's favour all manner of unforeseen incidents, meetings and material assistance, which no man could have dreamt would have come his way.
> ~ *J. W. Von Goethe*

We all have mentors and people who have profoundly influenced us: family, colleagues, role models, children. We also learn from the experience of others. Their *Pearls of Wisdom* have been invaluable. Observing, debating, challenging, laughing and sharing with them. We thank them, for we would not be who we are without them.

Assignment One

Applying The Bullets To Your Life

This book can be a tool if one applies the wisdom shared within. It can foster great change for you. Bulleted points at the end of each chapter can be applied to your life by asking questions, such as: what, why, how, who, where, when?

In this assignment, work on each bullet and apply it to your life by asking questions.

- What does it mean?
- What might be next?
- How does that apply to me?
- How can I implement it?
- Where would I implement it – home, work, play, family, parenting, financially, socially, community, physically, spiritually?
- Who do I need to become to achieve this?
- Where do I go from here?
- What would be my priority?
- What can I begin now?
- Why does this resonate with me? Or why does this bullet bother me?
- Where am I in comparison to where I want to be?
- What small step can I take now to move forward?
- Who can support me in making change?
- Do I need other information to make something change?

If you applied the bullet, how would things change for you? What would you accomplish? What would your life look like? How will you feel?

To implement further life enhancing strategies, see page 286!

Example 1:

What does it mean to you that, *you are the company you keep*? When you look at who you spend your time with, are the relationships healthy? Do they foster growth? Do they challenge? Or are they the polar opposite? Are the relationships life giving and promoting or compromising? Do you need to change the people you surround yourself with? Does your response need to change? Do you need to place boundaries on certain relationships?

Example 2:

What does it mean that, *there are no failures only lessons?* How can applying this attitude of learning from failures impact your life?

To implement further life enhancing strategies, see page 286!

Assignment Two

Tolerations

When we stop to simply notice and be aware of our surroundings, we may feel people, places or things are draining us of our energy. An example, when you walk into a room where an argument preceded your entrance and you feel the energy in the air, stifling and thick. Or you look at your desk full of clutter and sigh, "I must get that cleaned up." Or worse, you have people who suck the force from within you like a vacuum; though you want to help, you dread having the energy pulled from your vitality.

Tolerations rob our attention and our vitality, serve as distractions and prevent us from fully being present. It is difficult to function at our full potential when these "things" get in the way. Yet we may have been *tolerating* them, without even recognizing their effect on us. Clear them away, and keep alive the vital energy within.

What would happen to your life if you address every energy? Those that drain your vitality, and those that feed your vitality.

In this exercise:
1. **List the items, behaviors, environment or people who rob you of your energy (write them all down, even if the list is longer than anticipated).**
2. **Prioritize this list, with the biggest 'robbers' first.**
3. **Next to each item on the list, write how it makes you feel.**

To implement further life enhancing strategies, see page 286!

4. **Then write out a solution for making a correction (break down the solution into realistic, mini-manageable and achievable steps with an appropriate time-line to complete the steps.**

5. **Work at removing as many items from the list as you can, one at a time.**

6. **Revisit this list on a regular basis to keep it current, as well as fresh in your mind.**

You may prioritize by means of working at your most pressing items first. Alternatively, you may want to start small, and address items that are easier to remove. By beginning small, and achieving the removal of the interference, it will lead to bigger steps in the future. In order to remove the draining item, it may mean you need to change yourself.

Example 1:

Drain: I know eating a lot of pasta and bread makes me groggy and it is draining my energy.

Adjustment: I may need to remove it from my menu.

Example 2:

Drain: My relationship with my friend is a distraction from my life purpose because she does not support me in my mission, and becomes angry when I say I can not go shopping with her because I am commitment to my goals. This is draining my vitality because she always needs a full explanation, and I end up making excuses that match her values instead of mine. Although I love here, it is sacrificing a part of myself to continue our friendship in this manner.

Adjustment: I may need to place boundaries around my relationship with her, and speak to her less frequently. Without emotion or confrontation, I will let her know how her reactions make me feel. I will ensure I am not changing the tone

To implement further life enhancing strategies, see page 286!

of my voice when I tell her. I will request that she stops asking me to go shopping during the hours she knows I have other obligations to fulfill. I will identify the specific *behavior* and tell her how it makes me feel. I will insist if her *behavior* does not stop, there is a consequence of limiting the contact I have with her. And if her *behavior* does not change, I will leave the friendship. I will separate who she is from the unacceptable behavior.

Example 3:

Drain: I have had an experience of a new patient coming into my office fuming about the traffic being awful, angry about having a bad day, and demanding to see the doctor (me) immediately. He is loud, obnoxious and verbally disrupting the staff at the reception desk. My boundary was hit when I overheard the confrontation from my adjusting room.

Adjustment: I came out, inquired about the challenges. I made a point that the tone and language was unacceptable in my office and it needed to stop. If he could not stop, he would be asked to leave and I would be happy to find him a colleague to see him. He had a choice to either sit-down quietly to complete the paperwork and I would be with him at the appointed time, or he could leave. (He stayed and later apologized for this outbreak.)

More Pearls and Assignments can be found on the website www.pearlsofwisdompandp.com.

To implement further life enhancing strategies, see page 286!

Dr. Liz's Personal Help

I am like you: I generate great ideas but do not always move myself forward on them. I have learned that when I hold myself accountable to someone else, I vastly improve my success at making desired outcomes reality.

⇒ How often do you read fabulous ideas but fail to implement one single thing? You may have all the information you need, but lack the knowledge of how to make it reality. I know this book will inspire you, however your desire and intention has to be combined with action in order to achieve results.

⇒ Would it be easier to make changes when involved in a supportive community, together strategizing ways for everyone to win?

⇒ Is it easier for you to make changes with like-minded individuals, all working on self-improvement?

⇒ Are you more likely to follow through when you commit yourself to a program?

⇒ Do you want a framework to continue to implement and practice *Pearls of Wisdom* in your Life?

⇒ If you implemented a minimum of 20 ideas from this book, how would your life change?

Take action now and sign up for the 20-week *Pearls of Wisdom* Teleconference Group Coaching Classes. This program moves you through "knowing" what you should do, to actually "practicing it" and living it.

www.pearlsofwisdompandp.com

My wish is for you to gain the most benefit from this wisdom. I support your success with an enrichment program. This 20-week *Pearls of Wisdom* Coaching System joins Teleconferences with a *Pearls of Wisdom Journal* available online as part of the coaching system. This is a step-by-step plan to help you!

Sign up today to take advantage of the online program while it is available:

www.pearlsofwisdompandp.com/coachingjournal

References & Works Cited

For the purpose of simplicity, resources cited in more than one chapter are noted only once.

Response-Ability

1. Branden. Nathaniel. *The Art Of Living Consciously: The Power Of Awareness To Transform Everyday Life.* Fireside/Simon and Schuster. 1999.
2. Gerber, Michael. *E-Myth Revisited.* Harper Collins. 1995.
3. Hawkins, David R. *Power vs Force: The Hidden Determinations Of Human Behavior.* Veritas Publishing. April 2001.
4. Hunt, Valerie V. *Infinite Mind: Science Of The Human Vibrations Of Consciousness.* Malibu Publishing, Co. 1996.
5. Lipton, Bruce. *The Biology Of Belief.* Mountain Of Love/Elite Books. 2005. www.brucelipton.com.
6. Murphy, Joseph. *The Power Of Your Subconscious Mind.* Prentice Hall Press, Published by The Penguin Group. Revised version: 2008.
7. Carlson, Richard. *Taming Your Gremlins: A Surprisingly Simple Method For Getting Out Of Your Own Way.* Harper Collins Publishers. 2003.
8. Csikszentmihalyi, Mihaly. *Flow: The Psychology Of Optimal Experience.* Harper Perennial. 1990.
9. Dispenza, Joe. *Evolve Your Brain: The Science Of Changing Your Mind.* Health Communications, Inc. 2007, www.joedispenza.com.
10. Dodge, Norman. *The Brain That Changes Itself: Stories Of Personal Triumph From The Frontiers Of Brain Science.* Penguin. 2007.
11. Palmer, BJ. *Palmer's Law Of Life.* Palmer School Press. Davenport Iowa. Volume XXXVI, 1958.
12. Prochaska, James, et al. *Changing For Good.* Collins Living. 2002.
13. Robinson, Ken. *The Element: How Finding Your Passion Changes Everything.* Viking-Penguin. 2009.
14. Stephenson, Ralph.W. *Stephenson's Chiropractic Textbook.* Palmer School of Chiropractic, Davenport Iowa. Volume XIV. 1927. http://theatlasoflife.com/2010/04/29/the-33-

principles-of-chiropractic-by-ralph-w-stephensen-d-c-ph-c/.

15. Talbot, Michael. *Holographic Universe.* Harper Collins. 1992.
16. *Chiropractic Fitness and Wellness Magazine:* www.cwfmonline.com.
17. Chiropractic Leadership Alliance: www.subluxation.com.
18. Chiropractic Pure and Powerful: www.pureandpowerful.com.
19. Dyer Wayne: www.drwaynedyer.com.
20. Dynamic Essentials: www.lifede.com.
21. James Carter DC: www.carteruniversal.com.au/.
22. International Chiropractic Association: www.chiropractic.org.
23. *New Beginnings*: www.newbeginningschiro.com.
24. Parker Seminars: www.parkerseminars.com.

It Is Not Just One Thing

25. Re-told by Joel Barker, *The Power of Vision,* 1990. Originally written by Loren Eiseley (1907-1977), *Unexpected Universe,* 1969.

Lessons in Being

26. Dr. John Demartini – *The Breakthrough Experience*™ www.drdemartini.com.
27. Byron Katie – *Loving What Is:* www.thework.com.
28. Anthony Robbins – *Date with Destiny*: www.anthonyrobbins.com.
29. Abraham-Hicks – The Law of Attraction/The Vortex: www.abrahamhicks.com.
30. Bill Esteb – The Conversation: www.patientmedia.com.
31. Chiropractic Leadership Alliance – Total Solution: www.subluxation.com.

Anything, Nothing, Everything

32. Foundation for Chiropractic Progress: www.f4cp.com.
33. "Improving Fertility with Chiropractic Care:" www.sdfertility.com/pdf/March2004.pdf.

34. *Holistic Chiropractic Care Family Building Magazine*, Volume 6, Issue #1, Autumn/NIAW. 2006.
35. Infertility Research makes national news: www.worldchiropracticalliance.org/news/behrendt.htm
36. "Infertility, Interference and Infertility:" www.jvsr.com.
37. *Infertility:* "A public Health Focus on Infertility Prevention, Detection, and Management." www.cdc.gov/ART/infertility/PublicationPG2.htm.
38. *The Role and Relationship of Chiropractic and Women's Health Issues:* www.jvsr.com.
39. *Women Behaving Badly?* http://women.webmd.com/features/women-behaving-badly.
40. Static and Dynamic Surface Electromyography (sEMG): www.subluxation.com.
41. Professional Football Chiropractic Society: www.profootballchiros.com.
42. Chiropractic And The American Rescue, "The Chiropractic Relief Effort at Ground Zero." www.jvsr.com.
43. Study Reviews, "Chiropractic Efforts At 9-11 Rescue Sites." www.worldchiropracticalliance.org/media/9-11.htm.
44. CA Press Release, "Chiropractic Tops Wire Service List." www.worldchiropracticalliance.org/news/topslist.htm.

We Live the Life We Imagine

45. *Well Adjusted*: www.welladjusted.me.

A Life of Service

46. Girls Gals Gurus, Inc: www.girlsgalsgurus.com.

Now Is the Time

47. Peter Pan Potential. Pamphlets, newsletters and e-education: www.drclaudiaanrig.com.
48. Generations: www.generations.com.
49. Plaugher, G. and Anrig, C. *Chiropractic Pediatrics.* William and Wilkins. 1997.

When Destiny Calls

    50. Lepien, Marvin A. and Lepien, Rose. *Life Before Life, The Journey Of The Soul.* International Health Publishing. 2009.

    51. Dr. Lepien, Rose. Aaragon Chiropractic: www.aaragonchiropractic.com.

Honoring The Voice

    52. International Chiropractic Pediatric Association: www.icpa4kids.com.

    53. *Pathways to Family Wellness Magazine*: www.pathwaystofamilywellness.org.

    54. I.C.P.A.- Research and Public Education Foundation: www.icpa4kids.org.

    55. Academy of Chiropractic Family Practice: www.chiropracticpediatrics.com.

    56. Holistic Pediatric Association: www.hpakids.org.

    57. *Mothering Magazine*, "Ask the Expert:" www.mothering.com/experts/meet.shtml.

Contributing Authors
~ Alphabetically ~

Elizabeth Anderson-Peacock B.Sc, DC

Dr. Liz has a degree in Biology and graduated cum laude from CMCC in 1986. She enjoys a highly successful career as a Chiropractor, leader, and mentor with an internationally known pediatric-family practice, and is a contributor to numerous committees such as examinations, peer assessment, complaints and clinical practice guidelines. She currently sits on the board of the *WCWC, YMCA of Simcoe/Muskoka*, and is the President of the *Academy of Family Practice*. She is a seasoned speaker with topics ranging from technical aspects of practice-life to motivation, making change and teambuilding. Dr. Liz is well known for taking academics and *making it real* for both colleagues and patients alike. Published in many journals and magazines, she is also the recipient of *CLA's* "Chiropractor of the Month" in September 1996, "Canadian Chiropractor of the Year" in 1998, *WCA* "Chiropractor of the Year" in 1999, *OCA's* "Heart and Hand Award" in 2005, and *WCWC* "Woman Chiropractor of the Year" in 2008. Additionally, she was honored as a "Fellow" of the *ICA* in the 1998 and is featured in *Women With Vision* in 2007. She enjoys life with an extraordinary husband and family in Canada. Dr. Liz and her products are available through www.drliz.ca. She is the co-founder of *Girls Gals Gurus Inc.*, a company connecting women to Vitalistic health and wellness principles (www.girlsgalsgurus.com). Dr. Liz can be followed on *Twitter* at: drlizap.

Claudia Anrig DC

Dr. Claudia continues with full-time practice for the past 29 years and is the founder of the first comprehensive pediatric program and community outreach, *Peter Pan Potential*. She also personally mentors chiropractors with a dream of growing their family wellness practice in the *Generations Coaching Program*. She is the past president and currently serving on the board of the *ICPA*, and is on the post-graduate faculty of many Chiropractic colleges. She received the "Chiropractor of the Year Award" for 1997 from the *World Chiropractic Association*, "Fellow" of the *International Chiropractic Association* (ICA) in 1997, and "Distinguished Service" from the *ICA* in 1998. Dr. Anrig's textbook, *Pediatric Chiropractic*, is the first of its kind and is the fastest selling textbook in Chiropractic history. If you think you're ready to make the shift to a wellness practice visit www.drclaudiaanrig.com/gen_survey.html and you can schedule a one-on-one call with Dr. Claudia to learn more.

Jennifer Barham-Floreani BS, B.Chiro., DC

Dr. Jennifer is a graduate from Royal Melbourne Institute of Technology with a double degree in Chiropractic and Applied Clinical Science. Dr. Jennifer has been dedicated to encouraging the 'health literacy' of families and is a published authority on pediatric health and holistic parenting. She is well known for her book *Well Adjusted Babies,* as well as her "Health Expert" contributions in television and newspapers. She was awarded both "Australian Chiropractor of the Year" and "Victorian Chiropractor of the Year." Since birth, Dr. Jennifer has been adjusted by her father. She became a Chiropractor along with four out of five siblings, and is also married to a Chiropractor, Dr. Simon Floreani. She and her husband founded Vitality Chiropractic – an award-winning Health and Wellness super clinic incorporating over 20 Allied Health professionals located in Melbourne, Australia. Dr. Jennifer has four children and she can be reached through www.welladjusted.me.

Madeline Behrendt BS, DC

Dr. Madeline Behrendt is an award winning Chiropractor connecting women to Chiropractic and Chiropractors to women. Her work travels the worlds of fashion, film, research, media, and policy. Dr. Behrendt is licensed in New York, New Jersey, and Idaho, and moves between the city, the shore, and the mountains.

Justine Blainey-Broker DC

Dr. Justine learned at an early age the price of holding a value and a vision. In standing up for her beliefs and five court cases later, the *Ontario Human Rights Code* was amended to remove legislated inequality in sports, and Justine hit the ice to play hockey with the boys. Dr. Justine continues to believe passionately in equality. Dr. Justine has spoken in Chiropractic, health and well-being, goal setting, goal getting and volunteerism at places such as *Hydro One, Region of Peel Hospital, Police, General Electric,* Universities of York and Toronto, *Unilever, Wal-Mart*, church groups and numerous schools. She is a member of a number of professional organizations, a leader and coach for *Fortune Management*, as well as a loving mother and wife.

Dena Churchill B.Sc, DC
Dr. Dena Churchill, based in Halifax, N.S., is a Chiropractor, speaker, consultant and author of the new book entitled *Divinity In Divorce, The Power in Gratitude & Love.* Her book explores how people going through divorce and other life crises can find healing, wholeness and wisdom. In addition, Dr. Churchill is a regular contributor to the health, fitness and lifestyle magazine *Optimyz*. Dr. Churchill is an expert in the relationship between mind and body health, and a writer and speaker known for her clarity, wisdom and humor. She graduated from CMCC in 1996 and holds degrees in biology and psychology from Memorial University. Dr. Churchill studied Acupuncture at Xi Yuan Hospital, China Academy of Traditional Chinese Medicine in Beijing, China. She is among 1,000 facilitators worldwide trained through the *Demartini Method® Facilitator Global Group.* Her media appearances include interviews on *CTV* and *CBC-TV.* She is the mother of two sons ages 12 and 8, has a brown belt in Kempo Karate, and has been practicing yoga for seven years. To learn more about Dr. Churchill and her work, visit www.drdenachurchill.com, or visit her on social media under her name.

Lise Cloutier DC
Dr. Lise Cloutier has been a highly successful Chiropractor in the Ottawa area for more than 15 years. Dr. Lise graduated from the CMCC in 1995 with clinical honors, and is fully bilingual. Thanks to her continuous pursuit of excellence and investing in her own personal growth and development, Dr. Lise is also a well-known speaker, coach and CA trainer in the Chiropractic world. Dr. Lise is extremely passionate about educating and inspiring her patients to be proactive with their health and to live a wellness lifestyle as she advocates with her spouse and two children. Additionally, Dr. Lise is certified in Chiropractic Pediatrics through the *ICPA*.

Lezlee P. Detzler BA, DC

Dr. Lezlee obtained her undergraduate degree from the University of Guelph and graduated with honors from the CMCC in 1984. After a one year associateship, she returned to her home town of Durham, Ontario where she spent the next nine years building a highly successful practice. After selling her practice in 1994, Dr. Lezlee's career has been as a locum Chiropractor. She has traveled to a number of countries around the world, including a locum stop in New Zealand. Other travels have brought her to Zanzibar, Africa with *Hands Across Borders* to provide Chiropractic care to the local community. Since 2003 she has been serving the profession on a regulatory complaints committee. In 2007, she was the recipient of the "Presidential Award of Excellence" by the CCO. Dr. Lezlee's zest for life is based on inspiring and empowering others to optimize their health and wellness and live a life of their dreams. Dr. Lezlee has an active lifestyle, enjoys world travel and a desire for raw and live foods. She is forever grateful to her partner Sue for her unwavering encouragement and love, her niece April, and her close friends and family for their support.

Pat Gayman DC

Dr. Pat has been coaching since 1998. She is also a consultant, a speaker and an author. She writes an "Attitude Adjustment" newsletter and maintains a small part time practice. She is on the postgraduate faculty of three Chiropractic colleges and is an Adjunct Professor, formerly Dean of Clinics at Life Chiropractic College West. Known as the "Chiro Mom" she is passionate and enthusiastically committed to living life to its fullest. She started young (great grand kids already) and is still going strong! She loves her husband, family, friends, Chiropractic and fun of all sorts.

Janice Hughes B.Sc, M.Sc, DC

Dr. Janice Hughes is a leader, a teacher, an author and a coach to thousands of professionals worldwide. Her unique style of leadership has represented an extraordinarily valued asset to those whose lives she touches. Her blend of intuition, practicality and incredible focus has made her a role model for all professional women. Translating the same skill-sets into her current key role, she is engaged in the new venture *Curemark LLC*, a start-up biotechnology company. *Curemark* has matured into a major force in the area of autism and other neurological disorders with an unmet healthcare need. Janice brings to her new work a sense of urgency for the children with autism, as well as the ability to work in an environment where convention meets the unconventional, at the crossroads of health, science and humanity. Her work at *Curemark* underscores her life in that: anything is possible, 'no' is only a two-letter word, and with good leadership and a great idea one can change the world. Janice is married to her husband David Boynton DC, and with their three children they live in Boulder, CO.

Rose Lepien BS, DC

A native of Germany, Dr. Rose Lepien came to the USA as an ex-change student, and returned later to make this country her happy home. She is a very loving mother and stepmother and a cherished friend to many. She has been working in the field of Chiropractic for 37 years as Chiropractic assistant, office manager, Chiropractic wife and since 1991 as a practicing Doctor of Chiropractic. Dr. Rose has a degree in Science from Cameron University, and her Doctor-ate degree in Chiropractic from Parker College of Chiropractic in Dallas, Texas. She is very active in the Chiropractic world, is a board member of the *World Congress of Women Chiropractors* and has served 3 years as moderator. She has served 9 years on the Board of Parker College – four as Chairman of the Board. She has a large, successful Chiropractic practice in Lawton, Oklahoma where she is greatly involved in her community. She received the "Chiro-practor of the Year" award from *Parker Seminars*, "Women Chiropractor of the Year" from *WCWC*, "Outstanding Women of Comanche County," "Women in Business Champion" of Lawton and the State of Oklahoma, and the "Dr. Jim Parker Founders Award."
She has recently published her late husband's book *Life Before Life, The Journey Of The Soul*. Loving service is her first technique. She loves God, her patients, her immediate family as well as her Chiro-practic family worldwide, and looks forward to continued service to humanity by touching and changing lives through Chiropractic for many years to come.

Wanda-Lee MacPhee B.Sc, DC

Dr. Wanda Lee is a Chiropractor, speaker/trainer, consultant, author and leader in the Chiropractic profession. She has been in practice in Nova Scotia, Canada since 1994 along with her husband. Dr. Andrew Kleinknecht. Her greatest achievement is her two fantastic children, Claire and Thomas. Dr. Wanda Lee is also the President and creator of *The Chiropractic AudioCoach*, an online and teleseminar training and coach selection resource for the Chiropractic profession worldwide. She has donated countless hours to the profession she loves by serving and leading both provincial and national Chiropractic organizations. Dr. Wanda Lee is an avid student and continuous learner deeply grateful for the opportunity to pay back and pay forward the gifts she has received. She can be reached at chiropracticaudiocoach.com.

Carol Ann Malizia DC

Dr. Carol Ann graduated from NYCC and furthered her specialization becoming a Certified Chiropractic Sports Practitioner, along with becoming a Certified Personal Trainer by the National Academy of Sports Medicine. She has maintained a full spectrum private practice in upstate New York with the emphasis on lifestyle and longevity programs. She is currently the Woman's Health Editor for a national magazine, *Chiropractic Wellness and Fitness Magazine*, with a readership of 8 million. To her credit, she has accepted the position of board member for the Foundation for Chiropractic Progress (www.f4cp.org). Dr. Malizia was named Chiropractor of the Year in 1996 by *The Master's Circle*, recognized by the *Girls Scouts of America* as a "Woman of Achievement" in 2001, named "Woman Chiropractor of the Year" by the *World Congress of Women Chiropractors* in 2005, and in 2008 received "Chiropractor of the Year" by *Parker Seminars*. Dr. Carol Ann is relentless in her vision to educate, empower and influence the lives of millions by inspiring them to make quality healthcare choices and fulfill their own purpose in life. She possesses a burning desire backed with energy and enthusiasm to make a difference in the lives of people worldwide that she has the privilege to touch. She is co-founder of *Girls Gals Gurus Inc.* with Dr. Liz (www.girlsgalsgurus.com).

Jeanne Ohm DC

A practicing DC in a family, wellness based practice since 1981. Dr. Ohm is an International lecturer on the topic "Chiropractic Care in Pregnancy and Infancy." She is a post-graduate Instructor for numerous Chiropractic Colleges and author of many papers on pregnancy, birth, children and Chiropractic. She is the founder of Makin' Miracles...Connecting Kid's n' Chiropractic, community outreach programs and tools to educate children and adults about the life saving benefits of Chiropractic (www.makinmiracles.com). In addition, Dr. Ohm is the Executive Coordinator and Board Member for the *International Chiropractic Pediatric Association*: Editor of *Pathways to Family Wellness Magazine, The Holistic Pediatric Association* and panel member of *Mothering Magazine*. Dr. Ohm is married to Dr. Thomas Ohm, Chiropractor. They have six children who have all received Chiropractic care since conception. They were all born at home and are living drug free, healthy lives (www.icpa4kids.com).

Denise Perron DC

Dr. Denise Perron earned her DC degree from Palmer Chiropractic College in the mid 1980s. She ran a successful high volume practice in Montreal, Quebec, Canada from 1986 to 2008. Since, her focus has been on international speaking engagements, as well as postural analysis and postural digitizing tools. Her postural expertise has given her many opportunities to further educate and discuss Chiropractic Principles and the importance of postural evaluations. Dr. Denise Perron has lectured in Canada, USA, and Japan on the clinical aspects of spinal biomechanics and posture as they relates to patient care and communication. Dr. Perron has over 10 years experience with postural evaluation systems and tools. Recently, Dr. Perron levereraged her experience with technology to bring to market a new innovative product called *SHATOBU*: *'the workout you wear,'* a revolutionary shaper that *SHApes, TOnes* and *BUrns* calories. Today, she works full time in Research & Developement with *SHATOBU* (www.shatobu.com) and contiues to lecture in Chiropractic.

Andrea Ryan DC

Dr. Andrea Ryan graduated from Life University in 2002. She worked in both Connecticut and New York, and currently practices in Barrie, Ontario with her husband, Tom. She has been published in the *Journal of Vertebral Subluxation Research* and is the founder of the *Sprout! Program* for parents who are interested in optimal health for their children. She co-founded the *Wholistic Moms* group in her city, speaks to numerous groups on Chiropractic, and wellness. She is the mother of two beautiful children who keep her busy and teach her new things each day. Dr. Andrea enjoys marathon running, and has completed half and full marathons – one within a year of the C-Section delivery of her daughter. Dr. Andrea can be reached at www.andersonchiropracticgroup.com.

Grace Syn DC

Dr. Grace eats, breathes and lives Chiropractic and has an English Bulldog named Atlas. Dr. Grace resides in Redondo Beach, California where she runs a beautiful 4,400 sq. ft. successful practice focused on integrative family wellness care. She educates many people including professional athletes in the *NFL, AVP, NHL* and *Olympics* to improve their strength, coordination, peak performance and quality of life. Her accomplishments in the health field impressively include: speaker for *CalJam* 2009 & 2010, current President of *California Chiropractic Association - LASW District*, Chiropractic Leadership Alliance (CLA) "Chiropractor of the Month" July 2005, Founder of *TechniquePros.com* and *Comprehensive Chiropractic Technique* (CCT), Technique instructor for the CCA, certified *MC2* instructor, and author of *SpinePower* (TBR in 2011). Dr. Grace offers DC Training Programs in Redondo Beach, CA. For more information, visit www.techniquePros.com.

Cecile Thackeray DC

Dr. Cecile is a senior coach and Chiropractic consultant of *DC Mentors' Advisory Board*. She is a graduate of Canadian Memorial Chiropractic College (1985) with a fellowship designation in paediatrics through the *ICPA*. By perfectly combining the elements of Chiropractic practice, coaching, and motherhood, with attention to her personal interests and values, she learned to give her utmost in all areas of her life. She has completed her Chiropractor consultant training and certification in behavioural and value analysis. She has a true passion for understanding people; both mind and body. This, in combination with her strong intuition and experience lecturing, will help to create and unfold the best you that you can be.

Marlene Turner BA, B.Ed., DC

Dr. Marlene holds a Bachelor of Arts in Psychology/Sociology and a Bachelor of Education in Sociology and Physical Education. She graduated from CMCC in 1981, earning her Doctorate in Chiropractic. She served on both the Board of Governors of CMCC and the Task Force to Study Philosophy at CMCC. She co-founded The Chiropractic Forum and has presented for *James Carter Associates*, the *Chiropractic Forum*, *Healing Hands* and many other Chiropractic organizations. She was the instrumental voice of change in the local District School Board, where the policy for home education of non-vaccinated students was instituted in 1993. She practices in a beautiful century-old Victorian home in the Historic Downtown Milton, Ontario, Canada, and is blessed to be adjusting many of her patients from 1981 who continue as patients to this day. As a mother of four, Dr. Turner demonstrates it is possible to raise a family and run a very successful practice at the same time. She receives her inspiration from her friends and colleagues, and of course, her four children, Jonathan, Richard, Alisha and Mitchell.

Join and Connect

Your feedback and comments are encouraged and welcomed. Additionally, you may have a story that is important to share. With comments, feedback, and stories, please write to us at info@pearlsofwisdompandp.com. For information on further book study assignments for personal development and group study, visit www.pearlsofwisdompandp.com.

Other ways to connect:
Web: www.pearlsofwisdompandp.com
Email: info@pearlsofwisdompandp.com
Facebook: Elizabeth Anderson Peacock
Twitter: twitter.com/drlizap

For further information on coaching, women's seminars, workshops and retreats, and booking Dr. Liz Anderson-Peacock for your next event, write to info@pearlsofwisdompandp.com.

Order additional copies or bulk orders direct online
www.pearlsofwisdompandp.com
(List prices do not include shipping and handling.)

Dr. Liz Anderson-Peacock
c/o *Pearls of Wisdom, Pure & Powerful*
300 Lakeshore Drive, Suite 202
Barrie, ON L4N 0B4 Canada

Books also available through Amazon.com and InternationalHealthPublishing.com.

INTERNATIONAL HEALTH PUBLISHING

Inspiring readers of the world to experience the light.
International Health Publishing books express truth and wisdom,
encourage spiritual enlightenment, facilitate growth and healing –
while also providing a phenomenal reading experience.

International Health Publishing's vision is to increase the number and
quality of books and resources available to the public,
students and Doctors of Chiropractic – allowing for greater understanding, increased education, as well as more visibility and
accessibility of the Chiropractic profession as a means of
preventative and continued health care.

INTERNATIONAL HEALTH PUBLISHING
Adjusting and Growing
International Headquarters • Carrollton, Texas

www.InternationalHealthPublishing.com